To Bill, Wi

Reviews

"The growing crisis in long-tei   , .. ,ו.... Geyman describes, seems almost insurmountable, but, as he explains, it doesn't have to be so. Although it will test our nation's dedication to solidarity, we can ensure that we each have the best quality of life attainable under the given circumstances in our infirm years in spite of the trying circumstances that many of us will face. In "Long-Term Care in America," John Geyman tells us what can be done to help ease the tasks and tribulations for us and our caregivers."

—Don McCanne, M.D., family physician, senior health
policy fellow and past president of Physicians for
a National Health Program (PNHP)

"As the long predicted demographic tsunami of seniors rolls over the United States, Dr. John Geyman has written yet another invaluable book - this time about the developing crisis in long-term care. Now a senior himself, Dr. Geyman continues to write prolifically about America's broken health care system.

Backed by extensive, persuasive and easily understandable data, he defines the exploding problem of providing compassionate and affordable long-term care for the millions of our loved ones and neighbors now entering senior status - a problem that is both urgent and neglected.

He knows what he is talking about. In his previous book, *Souls on a Walk,* he recounted his 15 year experience as the primary caregiver for his late wife as her Alzheimer's disease progressed.

Most important, Dr. Geyman describes how we, as individuals and as a society, have arrived here and what we can and must do - personally and collectively - to live the best lives possible as we age."

—Phillip Caper, M.D., internist with experience in
health policy since the 1970s, and past chairman of the
National Council on Health Planning and Development

"Dr. Geyman has written another outstanding book that pulls the curtain back for all to see how dysfunctional our health care system has become. This book in particular is timely and essential reading. Long-term care in the United States is an issue largely ignored by the media and policymakers, but it is one that ultimately touches every family. It is beyond absurd that millions of Americans, the elderly in particular, have to spend down to poverty before they can get the care they need. Dr. Geyman explains how we got in such a mess and what we can do about it."

—Wendell Potter, founder of *Tarbell* and author of *Nation on the Take: How Big Money Corrupts Our Democracy* and *Deadly Spin: An Insurance Company Insider Speaks Out on How Corporate PR is Killing Health Care and Deceiving Americans.*

"A slow-moving caregiving crisis is building that is defying piecemeal incremental reforms, however well-meaning. If we are not already giving or receiving care, we know a friend or family member who is giving or receiving care. As society ages over the next few decades, the numbers will be unforgiving as the prevalence of Alzheimer's and other dementias accelerates, and caregiver shortages worsen.

Dr. Geyman is among a growing number of advocates calling for a comprehensive, universal solution that addresses the needs of the many millions of current and future disabled older and younger adults, unpaid family caregivers, and undervalued personal care aides. Arm yourself with the facts, stories, and policy prescriptions in this important book."

—Henry Moss, Ph.D., Board Member, Physicians for a National Health Program – New York Metro Chapter and author of *The 2030 Caregiving Crisis: A Heavy Burden for Boomer Children*

"Dr. John Geyman has spent the last twenty years document-ing the corrupt political economy of our health care system. From Obamacare to Medicare Advantage to Trumpcare to the so-called Public Option – Dr. Geyman traces the history of the medical in-dustrial political complex smothering the will of the people. As he describes in this compassionate and comprehensive book – *Long Term Care in America* – "under corporatized health care programs, the story is always the same – private profits, no price controls, less affordable, less choice, worse care, more profiteering, and inade-quate accountability."

Now, things are changing. Single payer is rising. And just in time, Geyman is now out with his clarion call for boomers – with 10,000 of us turning 65 every day. As he points out, by the age of 85, the odds of developing cognitive decline with dementia approach 40 percent.

Who is going to take care of you? And who is going to pay?

This book is coming out at a time when hopefully that question will be answered in the political arena. Congresswoman Pramila Jay-apal (D-Washington) has introduced the best single payer bill in the Congress – HR 1384 – with 118 co-sponsors in the House. It is the only single payer proposal that covers all long term health services.

Read this book. And then go to your member of Congress and demand action on comprehensive and immediate single payer.

OK, boomer?"

— Russell Mokhiber, founder of Single Payer Action,
and editor/publisher of *Corporate Crime Reporter,*
a legal weekly based in Washington, DC

"Geyman clearly articulates the immense and underrecognized challenges in the nation's long-term care system. He also maps a vision for the future, defined by quality jobs for direct care workers and quality care for consumers."

— Stephen Campbell, Policy Research Associate at
Paraprofessional Healthcare Institute

The Corporate Transformation of Health Care: Can the Public Interest Still Be Served? (2004)

Health Care in America: Can Our Ailing System Be Healed? (2002)

Family Practice: Foundation of Changing Health Care (1985)

The Modern Family Doctor and Changing Medical Practice (1971)

LONG-TERM CARE IN AMERICA

The Crisis All of Us Will Face in Our Lifetimes

John Geyman, M.D.

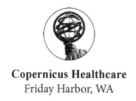

Copernicus Healthcare
Friday Harbor, WA

Long-Term Care in America
The Crisis All of Us Will Face in Our Lifetimes

John Geyman, M.D.

Copernicus Healthcare
Friday Harbor, WA

Ingram Edition
Copyright ©2020 by John Geyman, M.D. All rights reserved

Book design, cover and illustrations by W. Bruce Conway
Cover image used under license from Shutterstock.com
Author photo by Anne Sheridan

softcover: ISBN: 978-1-938218-25-5

Library of Congress Control Number: 2019919277

Copernicus Healthcare
34 Oak Hill Drive
Friday Harbor, WA 98250

www.copernicus-healthcare.org

Dedication

To the more than one-half of U. S. seniors expected to need long-term care in their later years, and to the more than 60 million Americans coping with one or more major disabilities, may you get the help you need, when you need it, that is affordable and fits your own personal situation. And to the dedicated caregivers who labor on without deserved compensation and recognition. And to the many activists, organizations, and elected officials working to restore comfort and dignity to the care that all of us will at some time need. May a better day be coming when system reform brings high quality long-term care that draws families and generations together in the later stages of their lives, and brings about a more vital national conversation about living and dying in our society.

LONG-TERM CARE IN AMERICA:
THE CRISIS ALL OF US WILL
FACE IN OUR LIFETIMES

CONTENTS

PART III: WHAT CAN BE DONE?

TABLES AND FIGURES

ACKNOWLEDGMENTS

As with my previous books, I am again indebted to many for making this book possible. Thanks are due to many health professionals, investigative reporters, and others for their probing reports on the status and shortfalls of long-term care in this country and our increasingly dysfunctional health care non-system. Especially helpful have been reports from the Kaiser Family Foundation, the Paraprofessional Healthcare Institute National (PHI), and Dr. Don McCanne's Quote of the Day (don@mccanne.org). Reports from many other organizations have also been useful in documenting the status of long-term care in the U. S., including the Center for National Health Program Studies, the Center for Disease Control and Prevention (CDC), the Centers for Medicare and Medicaid Services (CMS), the Commonwealth Fund, the Congressional Budget Office (CBO), the Office of Inspector General, Public Citizen, and the U. S. Government Accountability Office.

Special thanks are due to Paula Span, author of the excellent book, *When the Time Comes: Families with Aging Parents Share Their Struggles and Solutions,* for granting permission to reprint important questions to ask when considering various alternatives for long-term care. These are included in Appendix 1.

W. Bruce Conway, my colleague at Copernicus Healthcare over many years, has once again done a great job from start to finish of this book, including cover design, interior layout, typesetting, and conversion to e-book format. Carolyn Acheson has created a useful, reader-friendly index.

Many thanks are due to my eight colleagues who read advance copies and contributed generous comments as brief reviews. Most of all, I am grateful to my wife, Emily, for her careful reading and suggestions through many drafts of the book, including editing, proof reading, and promotion of the final book.

PREFACE

Providing personal and compassionate long-term care for aging seniors and people with disabilities has been a challenge over the last 100 years in this country. It has become much more of a challenge in recent years for a number of reasons, including its unaffordability even for well-off families, the lack of insurance to cover its costs, the aging of our population with increasing prevalence of dementia, mobility within families, the large number of people with disabilities, and the critical shortage of caregivers.

The markers of a growing crisis in long-term care are stark— by 2035, U. S. seniors over age 65 will outnumber, for the first time in our nation's history, the number of children under age 18; the odds of developing dementia by age 85 are approaching 40 percent; more than one-half of U. S. seniors are expected to need long-term care (LTC) help with activities of daily living in their later years; and one in four Americans has some type of disability, most commonly with mobility, cognition, and/or being able to live independently.

Despite this looming crisis in long-term care, we still have no national plan to make it accessible and affordable. Long-term care insurance has become a relic of the past, Medicare provides little coverage, and Medicaid only covers some costs after the patient has spent down to a poverty level.

What to do about the U. S. health care system was a big issue in the 2016 election cycle, and promises to be even more so as the 2020 election campaigns battle it out over future health care. It is an open question whether or not most of us will be able to afford long-term care when we need it, whether for our parents, our children, or ourselves. Will there be a safety net for us when we get there?

This book examines, in three parts, the big, largely unaddressed challenge of long-term care: Part I: What are the problems?; Part II: How did we get here?; and Part III: What can be done?

The U.S. remains an outlier among almost all advanced countries without a system of universal coverage of health care. It is my hope that this book will help voters and legislators to better understand policy alternatives, and to support what will best meet the needs of all of us for the care that we will all need, sooner or later.

—John Geyman, M.D.
Friday Harbor, WA
January, 2020

PART I

WHAT ARE THE PROBLEMS?

CHAPTER 1

INCREASING NEED FOR LONG-TERM CARE

Providing personal and compassionate long-term care (LTC) has been a challenge in this country over the last century, and is even more problematic today. As it becomes ever more unaffordable, even for well-off families, it puts many individuals and their families in a difficult bind as to how to care for their aging or vulnerable family members.

This chapter has three goals: (1) to discuss the major ways in which the need for LTC is growing exponentially in the United States; (2) to describe who pays (or doesn't pay) for the spiraling costs of LTC; and (3) to consider how we still lack a national health policy for providing LTC.

Factors Increasing the Need for LTC

They are multi-dimensional, dealing with demographic trends, clinical/health policy, socioeconomic and cultural factors in our changing society. These seem to be the most important that raise the stakes for providing compassionate LTC in this country.

Aging of the Population

According to a Population Reference Bureau report in 2016, the number of Americans ages 65 and older is projected to more than double from 46 million then to more than 98 million by 2060, with that group's share of the total U. S. population increasing from 15 percent to almost 24 percent. [1] Baby boomers, born between 1946 and 1964, are reshaping America's older population.

By 2035, U. S. seniors will outnumber, for the first time in our nation's history, the number of children under age 18. Figure 1.1 shows the magnitude of this ongoing change to the year 2050. [2]

FIGURE 1.1

SHARE OF OLDER POPULATION (65 YEARS AND OLDER) IN THE TOTAL U.S. POPULATION FROM 1950 TO 2050

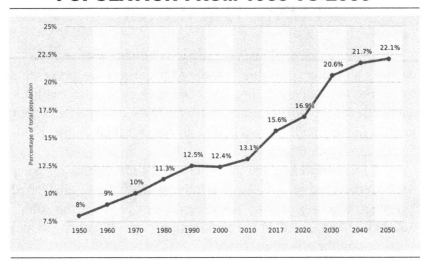

Source: U.S. Census Bureau and Statista, 2019

Length of Long-Term Care Needed by Nation's Seniors

More than one-half of U. S. seniors are expected to need nursing home or other LTC services in their later years, as shown by Figure 1.2. [3] These numbers raise the difficult question—what safety net can seniors depend on when people are living longer and health care costs become unaffordable on their fixed incomes? Social Security, under continued attacks by Republicans to cut the federal deficit, provides 90 percent of the income for one-third of the elderly and a majority of the cash income for more than 60 percent of seniors. [4] Meanwhile, public employers are cutting retiree health benefits and shifting to health reimbursement accounts (HRAs) that retirees can use as partial payment toward private insurance. [5] HRAs will not benefit the retirees, without the money to put into these accounts, and won't help toward the high premiums that insurers would charge for seniors with pre-existing conditions and likely several chronic diseases.

FIGURE 1.2

LENGTH OF LONG-TERM CARE NEEDED FOR U. S. SENIORS

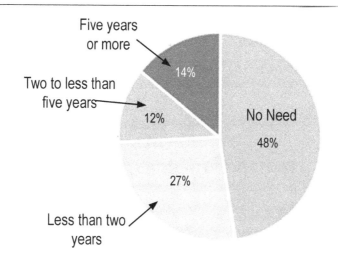

Source: Department of Health and Human Services

Probabilities of Illness and Disabilities for Aging Adults

In their important 2014 book, *Social Insurance: America's Neglected Heritage and Contested Future*, Theodore Marmor, Jerry Mashaw and John Pakutka identify six threats that separately or collectively threaten the ability of aging adults to cope with their changing circumstances. Table 1.1 summarizes the likelihood and consequences of any of these threats to be realized over the lifetimes of individuals. [6] Any one of these can obviously raise the odds that they will need LTC earlier and over a longer period of time.

TABLE 1.1

THE SIX THREATS

Threat	Probability	Consequences
Birth into a poor family.	25%-30%	At greater risk for violence, poor health, school dropout, incarceration, economic immobility.
Ill health		
Cancer	10% working life	Medical bills of $25,000-$100,000+, greater risk of death or disability
Heart disease	10-20% working life	Medical bills of $10,000-$100,000+, greater risk of death or disability
Early death	10% working life	Reduced family income by 50%-100%, greater child care expenses
Total disability	5%-10% working life	Reduced family income by 50%-100%, greater health care expenses
Involuntary unemployment	90% of one or more spells	Reduced family income by 33%-100%, increased risk of losing home, health insurance
Outliving one's savings	45%	Loss of independence, risk of becoming a ward of the state

Source: Theodore R. Marmor, Jerry L. Mashaw, John Pakutka, *Social Insurance: America's Neglected Heritage and Contested Future*, 2014, p.32

The number of disabled Americans is higher than we might expect. According to the Centers for Disease Control and Prevention, 61 million people in the U. S. (26 % of adults) live with one or more major disabilities that may make independent living no longer possible. Figure 1.3 breaks these disabilities down by type.

FIGURE 1.3

PERCENTAGE OF ADULTS WITH FUNCTIONAL DISABILITY TYPES

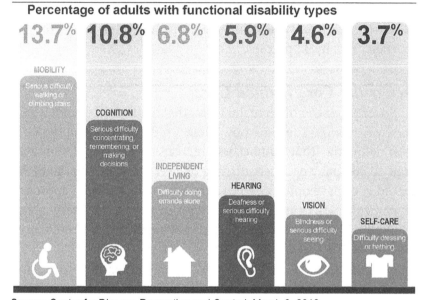

Source: Center for Disease Prevention and Control, March 8, 2019

When we look across our population by age group, we find that all of us are vulnerable to disabilities regardless of age:

- 2 in 5 adults age 65 and older have a disability.
- 1 in 4 adults age 45 to 64 with disabilities did not have a routine check-up in the last year.
- 1 in 3 adults age 18-44 with disabilities had unmet health care needs in the last year. [7]
- The prevalence of developmental disabilities increased among U. S. children age 3 to 17 between 2009 and 2017. [8]

Recent studies have found that early retirement is in itself also a risk factor. Early retirees may leave the work force at age 62, but experience an increased five-year mortality rate when they do so, together with a financial hit since Social Security replaces only about 40 percent of a typical paycheck. Early retirees often lose the mental stimulation of their work environment, become socially isolated, smoke and drink more, and start cognitive decline. Men who delay retirement in their early 60s lower their five-year mortality risk by 32 percent. [9]

Dementia: Care Without Cure

Dementia is another major factor that requires LTC somewhere and by someone. There are now some 5 million people in the U. S. with dementia. That number will increase as the population ages with 10,000 baby boomers turning 65 every day. By the age of 85, the odds of developing cognitive decline with dementia approach 40 percent. [10] The care of patients with dementia now costs about $200 billion a year, including actual payment for care and a large amount of unpaid care. [11]

The biggest risk factor for developing dementia is advancing age. As cognitive decline increases, the diagnosis is often missed. Those who receive a diagnosis are typically labelled with Alzheimer's disease, despite there being other kinds of pathology, including damage from physical trauma, strokes, diabetes, and other wear and tear of a long life. [12] Despite the hype from the pharmaceutical industry, there is still no cure for dementia. Care becomes the main strategy for dealing with this growing population.

Increased Inequality

The gap between the rich and poor in America has been in-creasing markedly over the last 50 years. As health care costs continue to escalate, more Americans can no longer afford care, leading many to delay or forgo it altogether. With incomes of middle class and poor Americans stagnant, one half of them face the choice of debt or care as collection agencies boom. Those who go without care experience worse outcomes. As one example of this widening gap, the wealthiest American men live 15 years longer than their poor counterparts. [13]

Increasing Disparities

Disparities have been increasing in the U. S. as the population becomes more heterogeneous in our dysfunctional, profit-driven system. These disparities occur across many dimensions, including race/ethnicity, socioeconomic status, age, location, gender and disability status. With less access to affordable care, disadvantaged groups have a higher burden of illness, injury, disability and mortality compared to their more advantaged counterparts. As just one example, low-income adults in Alabama are almost seven times more likely than high-income people to report skipping needed care because of cost. [14] Unless and until health care reform can address how care is financed, we can expect disparities to further increase as the population becomes more diverse.

International Comparisons of Long-Term Care

Despite being covered by Medicare, U. S. seniors face more financial barriers to health care, and are sicker than their counterparts in 10 other high-income countries. Across all these countries, almost one-quarter of U. S. seniors are considered "high need," in that they have three or more chronic conditions or require help with basic tasks of daily living. Nearly one-third of these patients skip care because of costs, compared to only 2 percent in Sweden, where universal coverage of health care was enacted many years ago. [16]

Who Pays for the Increasing Costs of Long-Term Care

About $300 billion is spent on LTC each year in the U. S., with Medicaid accounting for more than one-half of that number. Our current system is biased in favor of nursing home care over home and community-based services, although nursing homes are more expensive. That is because state Medicaid programs are required to cover institutional services, such as nursing homes. A number of states are getting waivers to cover home and community-based services, which are now becoming more available in some states. Nursing home care over a year costs more than twice as much as having a home health aide for a year and five times as much as the yearly costs of adult health day care. [16]

Regardless of any waivers, before they are eligible to receive LTC under Medicaid, patients must prove they are already in poverty or spend down their assets until they are in poverty. Medicare does not help much for LTC, since it covers only *short-term* rehabilitation in a nursing home. Indeed, our current national policy for LTC coverage drives large numbers of U. S. seniors into poverty. In her excellent new book, *Dementia Reimagined: Building a Life of Joy and Dignity from Beginning to End*, Dr. Tia Powell, professor of psychiatry and bioethics at Albert Einstein College of Medicine, observes:

> *This policy is a perversion of the Shakespearian adage: Some are born poor, some become poor, and some have poverty thrust upon them. We encourage elders to become poor, and if that doesn't work, we thrust poverty upon them.* [17]

Even when patients needing LTC are well off, they can end up in or near-poverty, as this patient's story illustrates:

> *Dr. S. played college football at Columbia University, after which he was recruited by the Chicago Bears. He negotiated an agreement whereby he could attend dental school while on the team. He helped the Bears win three championships, then switched over to dentistry. He developed dementia in his older years. His family kept him at home, where he had a team of workers, two for the day shift and two at night. In addition to Medicare, he had a Blue Cross supplement, together with a settlement from the NFL that gave him about $100,000 a year toward the end of his life. When he died at 97 as the oldest Chicago Bear, he almost qualified for Medicaid.* [18]

More than one-half of U. S. seniors are expected to need nursing home or other LTC services in their later years. Since the cost of LTC often exceeds $100,000 a year, most insurers are shying away from offering long-term care coverage as they encounter a growing frequency and duration of claims.

Ongoing Lack of a National Health Policy for Long-Term Care

In her excellent book, *Never Say Die: The Myth and Marketing of the New Old Age*, Susan Jacoby has this to say about the incoherence and shortcomings about how we deal with aging in this country:

> *The two overwhelming problems of real old age in the United States today are health, which generally worsens over time, and the tendency of all but the richest Americans to grow poorer as they grow older. Within these broad categories lie a host of specific issues that can be addressed only through collective action. A short list would include:*

> • *Medicare bias in favor of high-tech and surgical procedures instead of preventive health care. This bias discourages psychotherapy and ordinary doctor-patient consultations in which older patients might get a chance to talk about their health concerns instead of being hustled out the door with a new prescription. Medicare, as currently constituted, generally pays for a scan costing thousands of dollars but not for a fifteen-minute talk that might reduce the need for aggressive medical interventions.*

> • *The dearth of paid social services, provided at home or in community centers, that might keep many more of the frail elderly in their own homes and out of expensive assisted living facilities and even more expensive nursing homes.*

- *Failure to subsidize long-term care for those who need it and must therefor exhaust all of their assets before they can qualify for Medicaid, which generally provides the lowest quality of nursing home care for those who cannot afford to pay.*

- *A you're on your own government policy toward caretakers who want to keep family members in their homes but cannot bear the burden alone.*

- *A severe shortage, in many areas of the country, of affordable, accessible housing for healthy old people who have too much income to qualify for subsidies but not enough to pay market rate rents.*

- *Assisted living facilities are extremely expensive and not even needed by many older people whose disabilities are minor and whose needs might be better met simply by moving to an apartment—if they could afford the rents.*

- *Failure to use the skills of healthy old people who are able and willing to work either full-time or part-time— thereby easing their own financial burdens and continuing to contribute to society.* [19]

Family caregivers of developmentally disabled children, such as those with severe autism, are now elderly themselves as their middle-aged children face uncertainty about their future. Tens of thousands of these disabled adults, who have been at home their entire lives, are on long wait lists for state long-term care services in a system unprepared for their ongoing care. [20]

Under attack by deficit-minded Republicans, Medicaid is too leaky a boat to rely upon for the nation's LTC, especially as states' barriers for Medicaid coverage have been increased under the Trump administration. Moreover, given the enormous costs of LTC, it is unconscionable to rely on patients and their families to cover these costs. Medicare pays only about $11 billion of the $200 billion annual cost of dementia care, while care contributed by unpaid family members is by far the single largest source of care. [21]

How to pay for caregivers, after all these years, is still an unresolved question. They themselves are a vulnerable group—89 percent are women, most of whom women of color, with most uninsured, earning close to or below the minimum wage, without paid sick leave, and dependent on food stamps and Medicaid to support their families. [22] Though described by many as unskilled, their work is varied and hard. The care of frail and elderly patients, with or without dementia, often involves lifting patients who don't want a bath into and out of a tub, help with toileting, with many tasks potentially causing injury to the caregiver. Turnover rates in many home care agencies are more than 50 percent. [23]

There are many advantages to LTC being provided at home, which many patients and families prefer to institutional settings. But there are also many obstacles to such care. If home care agencies become involved, they typically take half of the hourly fee of caregivers, who take home less than $10 an hour. Home care workers have promoted a movement to increase the minimum wage to $15 an hour, which was opposed by many home care agencies. While home care workers do have the same protections for minimum wage and overtime as fast-food workers, they are pushing to unionize to obtain benefits, training, and more worker protections.[24]

As in other parts of our health care system, we urgently need to reform how we pay for health care. We will discuss this further in Chapter 10, where we make the case that single-payer Medicare for All is the *only* sustainable way of assuring universal coverage to affordable health care for all U.S. residents. Public Citizen, a strong advocate for Medicare for All, has this to say as it relates to LTC:

> *Instituting a Medicare for All system would offer an excellent opportunity to improve our approach to providing long-term care. These reforms would improve the quality of life of patients that need long-term care while also bringing down the cost of care, both for consumers and for the country as a whole. . . The long-term care benefits avail-*

able under Medicare for All should be designed to provide more comprehensive and sensible benefits than Medicaid, including ensuring that beneficiaries could be served in the setting of their choice. [25]

Conclusion

Having introduced ourselves to the problems of access and affordability of LTC, including the challenges of providing care to frail elders with dementia, we turn to the next chapter to discuss the many ways in which options to essential compassionate care are being reduced within our present under-reimbursed non-system of LTC. Meanwhile, the urgency of developing and implementing a national policy for LTC is well conveyed by Dr. Powell, who understands so well the high stakes involved:

Right now we have a big ugly hole in our health care policy. The problem for paying for dementia care is heading like a meteor toward the children of the baby boomer generation. We need to fix this, and soon. The current administration isn't even looking at the problem, but that won't make it go away. [26]

References:

1. Mather, M. *Aging in the United States*. Population Reference Bureau Report, January 13, 2016.
2. U. S. seniors as a percentage of the population, 1950 to 2050. *The Statistics Portal*.
3. Department of Health and Human Services.
4. Vanden Heuvel, K. Voters must catch on to Republicans' con on health care. *The Washington Post*, October 24, 2018.
5. Farmer, L. As retiree health care costs soar, public employers turn to private insurers. *Governing*, January 9, 2019.
6. Marmor, TR, Mashaw, JL, Pakutka, J. *Social Insurance: America's Neglected Heritage and Contested Future. Sage/CQ Press*, 2014, 31-32.
7. Disability and health. Disability impacts all of us. Atlanta, GA. Centers for Disease Control and Prevention, March 8, 2019.
8. Zablotsky, B, Black, LI, Maenner, MJ et al. Prevalence and trends of developmental disabilities among children in the United States, 2009-2017. *Pediatrics* 144 (4), October 1, 2019.
9. Johnson, RW. The case against early retirement. *Wall Street Journal*, April 22, 2019: R1.
10. 2017 Alzheimer's Disease Facts and Figures. Alzheimer's Association, 2017.
11. Hurd, MD, Monetary cost of dementia in the United States. *N Engl J Med* 368 (14), 1326-1334, 2013.
12. Powell, T. *Dementia Reimagined: Building a Life of Joy and Dignity from Beginning to End*. New York. *Penguin Random House,* 2019, 104.
13. Himmelstein, DU, Woolhandler, S. Health care inequality on the rise. *Huffington Post*, August 6, 2017.
14. 2018 Scorecard on State Health System Performance. New York. *The Commonwealth Fund*.
15. Osborn, R, Doty, MM, Moulds, D et al. Older Americans were sicker and faced more financial barriers to health care than their counterparts in other countries. *The Commonwealth Fund*, November 15, 2017.
16. Reaves, E, Musumeci, MB. Medicaid and Long-Term Services and Supports: A Primer, *Kaiser Family Foundation*, December, 2015.
17. Ibid # 12, pp. 176-177.
18. Ibid # 12, p. 169.
19. Jacoby, S. *Never Say Die: The Myth and Marketing of the New Old Age*. New York. *Pantheon Books*, 2011, pp. 272-273.
20. Goldberg, D. The health care system isn't ready to replace aging caregivers. *Politico*, November 13, 2019.

21.   Ibid # 18.
22.   *U. S. Home Care Workers: Key Facts* (2019) Paraprofessional Healthcare Institute (PHI) National. (2019), September 3, 2019.
23.   Ibid # 18.
24.   Ibid # 12, p. 175.
25.   *The Case for Medicare for All.* Washington, DC, *Public Citizen,* February 4, 2019.
26.   Ibid # 12, p. 185.

CHAPTER 2

A CONFUSING ARRAY OF OPTIONS FOR LONG-TERM CARE

As we saw in the last chapter, the need for LTC care continues to increase in the U. S. While it might seem that patients and families have plenty of options to consider when they have to decide on one path or another, there are many barriers to such choices, especially being able to afford care over a necessary period, or in many cases not having a full range of options available nearby.

As we all know, the need for LTC can arise quickly without much time to prepare for it, or more gradually as patients become less mobile and otherwise become unable to care for themselves. When either occurs, family resources are tested, including the ability to pay for care.

This chapter has two goals: (1) to briefly summarize the pros and cons of the main potential options for LTC, many of which may not be available in one's community; and (2) to discuss how patients and families can decide upon one option or another.

Pros and Cons of Potential Options for Long-Term Care
Home care

Many patients want to stay at home when they become disabled or need LTC, but that doesn't mean that it will be possible. How many family members will be available, and for how long, to provide such care? If more care is needed, will it be necessary to bring in paid caregivers, and can that be afforded? If patients with dementia start to wander, how can they be kept safe and how much more care will be required?

Demographic trends exacerbate this challenge. The divorce rate in couples has more than doubled over the last 20 years, and more than one-third of older divorcees live alone. [1] Baby boomers are aging alone more than any previous generation in U. S. history. About 8 million older Americans have no close kin. [2]

Many, if not most of us, would like to stay at home as we age with advancing chronic illnesses and disabilities, with or without dementia. As patients and their families deal with the possibilities, they need to develop a plan that is caring, affordable, and flexible enough to evolve through changing circumstances. That plan, of course, depends on available family support, finances, and available options in the community. This caregiver's story illustrates many difficult issues in coping with urgent needs for care within families across generations.

Alexis Baden-Mayer, now 45, moved with her husband and two children three years ago to take care of her parents at their home in Alexandria, Virginia. They put their own home on Airbnb to make the move when her mother developed Alzheimer's disease and was no longer able to care for her father with heart failure. In so doing, Alexis joined the army of some 34 million family caregivers in the U.S., mostly women, providing uncompensated care to frail elderly family members. As she says now, a frank conversation with her husband (not held in these blunt terms) would (or should?) have been: "What do you think about living with my parents for about ten years while their health declines and they die?" [3]

As a retired family physician, I was fortunate enough to care for my lovely wife Gene, at home, over what turned out to be a 16-year course with Alzheimer's dementia. From the start, home care was our first resort

We had been married for 40 years when Gene, at 61, first developed early signs of dementia. Subtle at first... We had a two-story house in the country, ten miles from town, and were able to stay there for almost 15 years. But by then she could no longer drive, was depressed and agitated, even delusional at times, and needed constant company after a near house fire that started on the stove.

It was time to move to a ground-floor condo in town. By then she was getting so confused that a frequent question in the middle of the night became "Where are we? Can we go home?" I put special locks on the door to prevent night-time wandering, but after she broke the door one night, that no longer worked. In the last 15 months, we finally needed around-the-clock care at home, and readily found a number of dedicated and caring home care professionals in our island community. We still wanted to avoid the local nursing home with its locked Alzheimer's ward.

Eventually Gene couldn't swallow and was hospitalized for the first time—4 days there in restraints with inadequate sedation (despite my efforts the whole time to convince the floor nurses and hospitalists of this problem), then 24 hours in an excellent hospice, where she was finally comfortable at the end. [4]

Although this did not result in burdensome debt, this experience does reflect growing burdens that finally required around-the-clock caregivers beyond myself. This 16-year course was difficult, heart-wrenching at times, but I treasure our joint journey together, and would have done it again the same way.

Although solo spousal caregiving at home during the last years of life is associated with increased depression and negative health outcomes for surviving spouses, a recent study found that 55 percent of spouse caregivers did so for their disabled spouses and even more for spouses with dementia. [5]

Families soon realize that caregivers are the key to a safety net, regardless of the location of care. Compared to earlier times, when families were less mobile and often stayed closer to their aging parents, it is now more difficult to start and sustain care at home by family members. One can seek paid caregivers through home health agencies or word of mouth from friends or others in the community. But these caregivers are often vulnerable themselves and it remains difficult to maintain ongoing help with such challenging problems as help with incontinence, mobility problems, disrupted sleep cycles, and behavioral problems.

Sometimes, home care ends up as a family's last resort, as this example shows:

> *Mrs. EF, 64, was working as a home health aide for seniors near San Ysidro, California, when she had to give up her job to provide the same care for her husband when he was recovering from triple bypass surgery. His health then declined as he developed vascular dementia with erratic behavior that caused her to fall and injure her back. He was admitted to one nursing home but later discharged because of his behavior. The local hospital was unable to find another place for him, so Maria brought him back home under her care.* [6]

Nursing home

There are about 15,000 nursing homes in the country, but that number is dropping as more close, especially in rural areas. Here is one such example among 440 closures of rural nursing homes last year:

> *Mr. L, 89, spent much of his life farming and ranching the rolling Dakota plains along the Missouri River. Late last year, the nursing home in Mobridge, S.D, announced that it was shutting down after a rocky history of corporate buyouts, unpaid bills and financial ruin. His town of 3,500 was too small to have a reservoir of home health aides for hire around the clock. His wife could not find any nursing home nearby that would take him, so he ended up in one 220 miles away in North Dakota, far from family, friends, and his roots.* [7]

Two-thirds of nursing homes are for profit, often in large chains. In recent years, private equity firms have found new markets of "serving" some of the nation's poorest and most vulnerable people—residents of nursing homes. They are in business primarily to make money for their CEOs and shareholders. They make big profits by pooling money from investors, borrowing even more, and then buying, revamping, and selling off nursing home companies.

Here is an example of a widespread national trend of evictions of patients that needed more care than nursing homes were willing to provide with their leaned-out staffs:

> *Mrs. S, 82, became more agitated with Alzheimer's and was discharged from a California nursing home where she lived with her husband. Although she won an appeal, the nursing home still would not accept her back. As her attorney said, "They don't take you back and there are no consequences.* [8]

Cutbacks in state Medicaid budgets are another cause of evictions from nursing homes, as occurred in Louisiana in 2018 when more than 30,000 Medicaid recipients in nursing homes and group homes were notified that they would face eviction due to proposed state cuts. [9] In March 2019, the Trump administration proposed a federal budget that would cut federal spending on Medicaid by $1.4 trillion and Medicare by more than $800 billion over the coming decade.

Assisted living

The overall goals of assisted living facilities are to provide 24-hour personal care and assistance in a homelike setting. They are community-based where the staff takes responsibility for the safety and well-being of an adult. Housing, meals, supervision, and various levels of care are provided, including help with activities of daily living, such as bathing, dressing, using the toilet, and taking medications. Some social and recreational activities may also be provided.

As with nursing homes, about 60 percent of assisted living facilities are for-profit, many owned by regional or national chains, with the costs and quality of care quite variable. [10] Assisted living is mostly a private pay situation without Medicaid coverage. While intended to serve an "aging in place" goal, assisted living facilities are more often where patients die or are moved along to nursing homes where they can receive more care.

Continuing Care Retirement Community (CCRC)

These are residential facilities that offer a range of housing options, typically from independent living to assisted living to nursing home care, and even hospice, in one community-based setting. People are often relatively healthy when they select this option. Upon entry, they sign a lifelong contract for either rental or ownership of their living space, and select their initial type of care.

Adult family home

These are regular neighborhood homes that can accept two to six residents, who will receive a room, meals, laundry, supervision, and varying levels of assistance with care. Some offer specialized care for patients with mental health issues, developmental disabilities, or dementia.

Adult day care

This is a supervised non-residential program that provides transportation, a meal, and a variety of health, social, related support services in a protected setting during the day. These services can help some patients with dementia to stay in the community while giving caregivers at home a break. Some adult day health programs may be available that provide counseling, skilled nursing and rehabilitative therapy.

Other community based services

A 2015 study of more than 15,000 providers across four categories—home care, adult health day care, assisted living facilities, and nursing homes—compared annual costs of LTC for these services. Figure 2.1 shows how much more expensive nursing homes are compared to these other categories. [11]

FIGURE 2.1

MEDIAN ANNUAL COSTS FOR
LONG-TERM CARE SERVICES (2015)

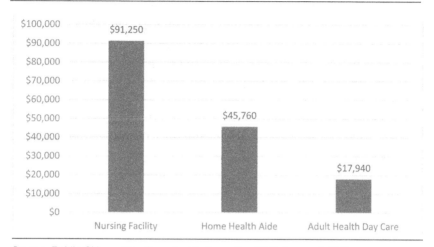

Source: Public Citizen: *The Case for Medicare-For-All*, February 4, 2019

Medicaid, the largest payer for LTC, accounts for more than one-half of the approximate $300 billion a year spent on LTC. As previously noted, a year of care in a nursing home costs more than twice as much as having a home health aide for a year and five times as much as a year of care through adult health day care. However, Medicaid's policies are biased in favor of patients ending up in nursing homes because it is required to cover institutional services, while home and community-based services are optional.

Because care in nursing homes is so much more expensive, a number of states have gained waivers of certain federal Medicaid requirements in order to expand access to some community-based services. As a result, LTC in home and community-based services recently overtook institutional coverage in terms of overall Medicaid spending for LTC. [12] Although this has been helpful, before Medicaid recipients can get LTC under Medicaid, they must first spend down their assets to poverty levels. Even then, there may be waiting lists before they can gain access to these other settings. [13]

Here are some of the important programs available in some states.

Family Caregiver Support program

The National Family Caregiver Support Program (NFCSP), established in 2000, provides grants to states and territories to fund various supports that help family and informal caregivers provide care for older adults in their homes for as long as possible. These types of services are provided:

- information to caregivers about available services;
- assistance to caregivers in gaining access to the services;
- individual counseling, organization of support groups, and caregiver training;
- respite care; and
- supplemental services, on a limited basis.

Studies have documented that these services can reduce caregiver anxiety, stress, and depression, thereby enabling them to provide care longer and avoid or delay the need for costly institutional care. [14]

Program of All-Inclusive Care for the Elderly (PACE)

This is an important program, first pioneering at the On Lok senior center in San Francisco, for people disabled enough to qualify for nursing home placement, but also are covered by both Medicare and Medicaid. This is a win-win for patients, families and government payers. The disabled elder gets to stay at home safely and happily, while expensive and unwanted nursing home care is avoided.

PACE programs, now expanded to 114 sites around the country, have been shown to decrease the use of hospitals and nursing homes as most participants improve or maintain function.[15] PACE also saves money through less use of such services as physical therapy day centers, primary care, and social work visits. [16]

Naturally Occurring Retirement Community (NORC)

This is a residential community not specifically designed for the elderly, but has a majority of residents over age sixty. Starting with the first NORC in a large apartment complex in New York City, they have now spread across the country connecting elders with services promoting health and social interaction. They tend to be in urban areas for residents with functional impairment and economic vulnerability, and to have paid staff with government funding. NORCs provide transportation to doctors' visits, coordinate with Meals on Wheels, arrange for outings, and provide exercise classes. Those services can make all the difference in allowing participants to remain at home and avoid nursing home placement.[17]

Village

The Village movement started on Beacon Hill, an affluent section of Boston, serving people who are financially more stable and have fewer functional impairments. They rely on volunteer service exchanges and are financed mostly by membership dues. There are now many such villages across the U. S. One example of their services is to provide a registry of discounted providers for home repairs. Both NORCs and Villages may organize grocery delivery for participants just home from the hospital, as well as encourage a range of social activities. While neither are designed for demented elders, they can help those with mild or moderate dementia delay or avoid nursing homes. [18]

How Can Patients And Families Decide Among These Options?

Many, if not most of us, would like to age in place if we are comfortable in our home and community setting. But that will require good planning in earlier years, as well as good fortune when the time comes for LTC.

For aging parents whose children have moved on with their lives elsewhere, an obvious place to start is the house or apartment itself. One-story houses are ideal, without multi-step entries (unless they could be ramped), with an extra bedroom for caregivers to sleep, hallways big enough for a wheelchair, and bathrooms with high toilets, easy entry tubs and protective hand bars. One may need to move from multi-story living before needing LTC.

Family and financial considerations are, of course, essential parts of a changing equation. Will any family members be available to help with LTC when it becomes necessary, and for how long? In many cases, volunteer or paid home health aides will be needed if family caregivers are not available. With the enormous costs of nursing homes, the goal would be to avoid that care for as long as possible. At the same time, paid caregivers providing LTC around-the-clock can also drain families' financial resources quickly. We can probably assume that few of us will have long-term care insurance, since that has become prohibitively expensive if it is even available at all in an industry that is going away.

As we saw above, other settings can provide aging in place, such as a CCRC or NORC. For many people, CCRCs are a good answer, but it takes sizable financial resources to buy in for a life-long contract and these facilities may not be available in one's community.

In the most common situation, we as individuals or as couples, have plenty of time to consider how to best deal with a future time when either or both of us will need LTC. Forward planning should include our health status and risk factors for disability and dementia, our financial reserves as we age, the proximity of other family members, and the availability of community resources for LTC. A move may become necessary to gain access to such facilities and/or to get closer to other, younger family members. Good cross-generation communication within the family is key to a good outcome for all concerned. See Appendix 1 for key questions to ask when exploring options for long-term care.

Day programs, if available in one's community, can be helpful in delaying need for caretakers in other settings. Being able to continue driving becomes another important factor.

Dr. Powell gives us good advice if and when we need to consider moving to an assisted living facility:

> *Look at how people live. Can they sleep and wake on their own schedule, or do they get roused rudely out of bed as in jail? Can they eat when they want, or will they miss breakfast if they don't get up on the facility's schedule? Some of the best places are not glamorous, but manage to create a real sense of community. If I go to assisted living, I'd like to stay there as I decline, and some places make that impossible. Others embrace the likelihood of change by offering different levels of care, including palliative care and hospice on site. I want to avoid the cycle of transfer from where I live, whether at home or in a facility, back and forth from the emergency department, the hospital, and home again.* [19]

Since falls as we get older are such a common cause notching us down functionally after a broken hip or other injury, we need to consider how best to avoid them. The most common site of these falls is in the bathroom, but others are often outside around our homes. A decision to wear some kind of a Life Alert can be very important if we fall alone and can't get up.

Hospice and Palliative Care

Many of us would like to avoid prolonged care that won't change our outcome, such as feeding tubes in a nursing home. Most of us also want to avoid unnecessary pain in our last days and months. Palliative care and decisions about hospice will prevent that if we think through and establish advance directives that are communicated to our family, physicians, and other caregivers. We will discuss this further in the last chapter. Useful resources on advanced directives are also included in Appendix 3 on page 184.

A physician's order is required to initiate hospice care, after which the goal becomes comfort for the patient's end of life care. Decision making about whether, and when, to shift over to hospice care, regardless of its location, poses a most difficult and stressful challenge to family members, physicians and other caregivers. Unless the patient has made clear his or her desires in an earlier advance directive, a family member with the power of attorney for health care often needs to clarify the patient's and family's desires. They need to recognize that Alzheimer's and the other dementias are progressive terminal diseases and that patients with advanced dementias are already near the end of life. At this stage, they have bladder and bowel incontinence, typically have a vocabulary of one word or less, and are dependent on caregivers for all activities of daily living, including walking, showering, and going to the toilet. Medicare coverage for this kind of care is based upon an expected duration of six months, but it is often difficult to estimate life expectancy for these patients.

Dr. Susan L. Mitchell, Professor of Medicine at Harvard Medical School and Director of Palliative Care Research at the Hinda and Arthur Marcus Institute for Aging Research in Boston, brings us this useful patient vignette as a decision aid in making the decision for comfort care:

An 89-year-old nursing home resident with a 10-year history of Alzheimer's disease presents with a temperature of 38.3 degrees C, a productive cough, and a respiratory rate of 28 breaths per minute. Nurses report that for the past 6 months he has been coughing at breakfast and having trouble swallowing. He has profound memory deficits, no longer recognizes his daughter (who is his health care proxy), is bedbound, is able to mumble a couple of words, and is unable to perform any activities of daily living. The nurse asks whether he should be hospitalized. How should this patient be evaluated and treated? [20]

In her excellent 2015 article in the *New England Journal of Medicine*, Dr. Mitchell gives us a caring and evidence-based approach to this question. As she points out, the patient probably has aspiration pneumonia, precipitated by swallowing problems that are common in advanced dementia and won't go away. Any further tests or treatments in the hospital would not alter his poor general prognosis. The advantages and disadvantages of treatment options should be outlined. If comfort measures are preferred, no further workup is indicated as palliative care goes forward for treatment of symptoms. [21]

Moving patients to hospice, whether at home, in a nursing home or at an assisted living facility, can bring personalized comfort care that can prevent needless trips to ERs or hospitalizations for acute problems that would just add discomfort and expense without changing the outcome of care.

Conclusion

What lessons can we learn about system problems that relate to possible solutions that will be further discussed in Part III? These come to mind:

1. Most of us can't save enough money to cover LTC, no matter how well off we are in earlier years.
2. The current system of LTC is volatile and too often unresponsive to our needs.
3. Poor care is common, including patient neglect and harm.
4. There is a need for greater accountability vs. profiteering and fraud in LTC facilities.
5. The costs of LTC put a growing strain on individuals and families' budgets, as well as Medicaid and Medicare budgets.
6. What safety net we still have is being shredded by current health policies that can be addressed through system financing reform.

Beyond options for places for LTC, it is now time to turn our attention in the next chapter to a major barrier to needed care—the increasingly unaffordable costs of care regardless of setting.

References:

1. Klinenberg, E, Torres, S, Portacolone, E. *Aging Alone in America.* Council on Contemporary Families. Austin, Texas, 2013.

2. Adamy, J, Overberg, P. More than ever, Americans age alone. *Wall Street Journal*, December 18, 2018: A1.

3. Gedye, F. The strange political silence on elder care. *The Washington Monthly*, July-August 2019.

4. Geyman, J. *Souls On a Walk: An Enduring Love Story Unbroken by Alzheimer's.* Friday Harbor, WA. *Copernicus Healthcare*, 2012.

5. Ornstein, KA, Wolff, JL, Bollens-Lund, E et al. Spousal caregivers are caregiving alone in the last years of life. *Health Affairs 38 (6): June 2, 2019: 964-972.*

6. Sanger-Katz, M. 1,495 Americans describe the financial reality of being really sick. *New York Times*, October 2017, p. 4.

7. Healy, J. Nursing homes are closing across rural America, scattering residents. *New York Times*, March 4, 2019.

8. Bernard, TS, Pear, R. Complaints about nursing home evictions rise, and regulators take note. *New York Times*, February 22, 2018.

9. KHN Morning Briefing, Thousands of nursing home residents face eviction due to Louisiana's cuts to Medicaid funding. *Kaiser Health News*, May 9, 2018.

10. Span, P. *When the Time Comes: Families with Aging Parents Share Their Struggles and Solutions.* New York. *Springboard Press*, 2009, pp. 115-116.

11. Reaves, EL, Musumeci, MB. Medicaid and Long-Term Services and Supports: A Primer. *Kaiser Family Foundation*, December 2015.

12. Eiken, S et al. Truven Health Analytics, Medicaid expenditures for long-term services and supports (LTSS) in FY 2015.

13. Ibid # 10.

14. National Family Caregiver Support Program. Administration for Community Living, March 26, 2019.

15. Fretwell, MD, Old, K. Zwan, K et al. The Elderhaus Program of all-inclusive care for the elderly in North Carolina: Improving functional outcomes and reducing cost of care: Preliminary data. *J Amer Geriatric Society* 63 (3): 578-583, 2015.
16. PACE, National Pace Association website, npaonline.org
17. Powell, T. *Dementia Reimagined: Building a Life of Joy and Dignity from Beginning to End.* New York. *Penguin Random House*, 2019, p. 179-180.
18. Greenfield, EA et al. A tale of two community initiatives for promoting aging in place: Similarities and differences in the national implementation of NORCs and Villages. *Gerontologist* 53 (6): 928-938, 2013.
19. Ibid # 17, p. 271.
20. Mitchell, SL. Advanced dementia. *N Engl J Med* 372: 2533-2540, 2015.
21. Ibid # 20.

CHAPTER 3

HIGH, UNAFFORDABLE COSTS OF LONG-TERM CARE

As the need for long-term care increases in the U. S., its increasingly unaffordable costs have become a major barrier for many patients and their families. This chapter has two goals: (1) to describe the main drivers of increasing health care costs in this country; and (2) to discuss the many ways that seniors, disabled patients, and their families encounter burdensome debt as they try to navigate options for long-term care within an increasingly shredded safety net.

Main Drivers of Soaring Health Care Costs

We now spend more than $3 trillion a year on health care in the U. S., more than $10,700 per capita. [1] Uncontrolled prices have been found to be the biggest driver in the spiraling costs of health care, with no cost containment on the horizon. Our profit-driven market-based health system has become corporatized and consolidated, with a small number of corporate stakeholders with large market shares charging what the traffic will bear.

Wall Street investors thrive as health care stocks lead the pack on the S & P 500 while patients and families—the reason for health care—suffer as they try to pay the bills for essential care. Because of the high prices, it has become the norm for patients to forgo or delay necessary care, then later have worse outcomes if they ever do get care. According to the Peterson-Kaiser Health System Tracker, one in ten adults either delayed or did not receive necessary care due to costs in 2016. Almost one in five U. S. residents do not fill a prescription each year because they can't afford them as the five largest pharmaceutical companies brought in more than $50 billion in profits in 2015. [2]

Here are some examples of outlandish prices as reported by the recently launched investigation by *Kaiser Health News* and *NPR* 'Bill of the Month:'

- Drew Calver's $109,000 bill for out-of-network care of his heart attack
- Shereese Hickson's bill for $123,000 for two new multiple sclerosis treatments, despite her being on both Medicare and Medicaid
- Benjamin Hynden's $9,000 CAT scan in an E.R., despite having had a similar scan just a few weeks before for $268 [3]

Bringing this down to family budgets, American households of four people now pay an average of $28,386 a year for insurance and health care, according to the 2019 Milliman Medical Index.[4]

Here are some examples of impacts on budgets of families, as illustrated by the medical bill score, as to how many of the public have taken these actions in order to pay their medical bills:

- 72 percent put off vacations, household purchases
- 70 percent cut back on food, clothing, basic items
- 59 percent used up most of their savings
- 41 percent took an extra job or worked more hours
- 37 percent borrowed money from friends or family. [5]

The continued escalation of health care costs is not due to increasing utilization of services, but to *unimpeded price increases* in an unsustainable corporate-run market. Figure 3.1 shows how prices and spending for health care have been increasing while utilization of some services, especially inpatient care, have been sharply declining due to costs. [6]

In the current deregulated environment, the medical-industrial complex makes it impossible to rein in the accelerating costs of U.S. health care. The health care industry spends at least $30 billion a year marketing its wares, driving more testing and treatments. [7]

FIGURE 3.1

CUMULATIVE CHANGE IN HEALTH CARE PRICES, USE, AND SPENDING, 2012-2016

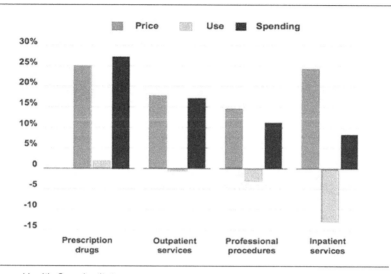

Source: Health Care Institute

Big PhRMA is a classic example of this problem. A 2018 report examined the price increases for the 20 most prescribed prescription drugs for Medicare Part D beneficiaries, including Crestor, Lyrica, Restasis, Symbicort, Tamifluu, and Xarelto. The prices went up by 50 percent between 2012 and 2017 for 12 of the drugs; for 6, they skyrocketed by more than 100 percent over those years. [8] The pharmaceutical industry maximizes its profits in a number of ways, including direct-to-consumer advertising (banned in many countries), non-rigorous "research" for marketing purposes, and lobbying against negotiated drug prices and importation of drugs from other countries.

Spending on health care in this country is projected to grow 1 percent faster than the GDP until 2026, when it will account for almost 20 percent of the U. S. economy, according to the Centers for Medicare and Medicaid Services. Figure 3.2 shows how the Consumer Price Index for medical costs has gone up exponentially over the last 40 years compared to the CPI. [9]

FIGURE 3.2

INCREASING BURDEN OF HEALTH CARE COSTS, 1980 TO PRESENT

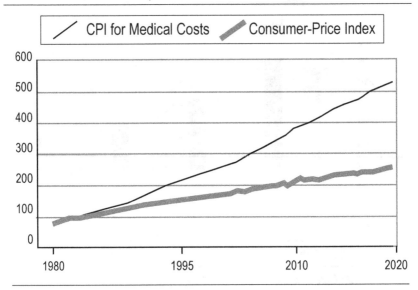

Source: Federal Reserve Bank of St. Louis

Ways in Which Seniors Can't Afford Long-Term Care

Facing these relentless increasing costs of health care, there are many reasons why seniors in America cannot afford needed long-term care.

1. Disadvantaged entry into retirement years

Seniors today enter their retirement years at a disadvantage for several reasons. The Affordable Care Act (ACA), enacted in 2010, did not control prices or costs. If they had employer-sponsored health insurance in their working years, they were finding higher cost sharing, with ever-increasing deductibles and co-insurance, and reduced benefits of their plans. [10] Even with the bull market on Wall Street since the recession of 2008 and 2009, investments in their pensions lost value. [11] Even as they needed more health care in their later years, they were paying more for less care because of the increasing costs of care. [12]

Two other factors will make it increasingly more difficult for seniors in their retirement years to afford LTC. First, the number of middle-income retirees with annual incomes in the $25,000 to $74,288 range today will more than double by 2029, when more than one-half of them are projected to have total financial resources of just $60,000 or less, even if equity in their houses is included.[13] Second, 37 percent of the average Social Security check now goes to their out-of-pocket health care costs. [14]

This situation is a constant worry for many people doing well now but facing future unaffordable costs of LTC:

> *Gretchen Harris, 72, a retired attorney, lives alone in her single-story brick house in Norman, Oklahoma, where she has practiced law for many years. Divorced, childless, and without family nearby, she still hears cases a few days each month as a state administrative law judge. She is dealing with multiple medical problems, including heart disease, non-Hodgkin's lymphoma, rheumatoid arthritis, and osteoporosis. She has no retirement savings and still has a mortgage on her house. Even after selling her house in the future, her income then will be about $4,600 a month from a state pension and Social Security. But the average cost of a one-bedroom apartment in assisted living is projected to use every bit of that in ten years, putting her in the classic "middle class bind." [15]*

2. Cutbacks in retiree benefits

Many states have promised hundreds of billions more for retiree health benefits than they have saved for that purpose. The gap in these post-retirement benefits is now about $600 billion, on top of the $1.4 trillion that states need to pay for promised pension benefits, according to the Pew Charitable Trusts. In response to this growing problem, some states are aggressively cutting retirees' benefits. North Carolina will end future retiree health care coverage in 2021, Kansas is asking retirees to pay the full cost of their health care, and Iowa has capped the contribution its flagship university makes to retirees' health care, cutting its liability by $465 million. [16] As the cost of medical care rises, states' promises to provide health care to their employees in retirement are growing increasingly unreliable.

3. Increasing out-of-pocket costs under Medicare and Social Security

Although traditional Medicare has been a solid rock in a stormy sea of the health care marketplace for many years, that rock is being eroded for the 59 million people so covered over age 65 and younger adults with permanent disabilities. A 2018 study from the Kaiser Family Foundation found that:

> "In 2013, Medicare beneficiaries' average out-of-pocket health care spending was 41 percent of average per capita Social Security income; the share increased with age and was higher for women than men, especially among people ages 85 and over; that percentage is projected to rise to 50 percent in 2030." [17]

Even with prescription drug coverage under Medicare Part D, beneficiaries typically face substantial out-of-pocket costs, especially for specialty drugs or multiple high-cost brand-name drugs.[18] A 2018 analysis of the 2016 Consumer Expenditure Survey documented that the financial burden for Medicare households has become more than double that of non-Medicare households (14 percent vs. 6 percent). (Figure 3.3) Nearly 3 in 10 Medicare households spent at least 20 percent of their total household income on health care in 2016, with this number increasing markedly with age. [19]

Social security is also being cut back, and is no longer a reliable source of funding for seniors on fixed incomes. This patient's story illustrates the problems even with an employer pension plan.

Mary Fry's husband, Virgil, worked in construction for 30 years, earning a pension of $3,568 a month on retirement, which was guaranteed to continue for Mary if he died first. Three years after his death from cancer, however, her payments were permanently reduced by more than one-half to $1,514 per month. Mary, age 72, who is a cancer survivor herself in western Ohio, could only say "It was quite a shock. It's worrisome, and I don't need to worry in my life right now. [20]

The cause of this indefensible action is the growing weakness of the U. S. pension system whereby "multiemployer" pension plans, which cover pools of union members working for different companies, are failing at an alarming rate. Unfortunately, this story will become common in future years, since about 12 percent of workers with vested multi-employer pensions are in plans expected to run dry within 20 years. [21]

FIGURE 3.3

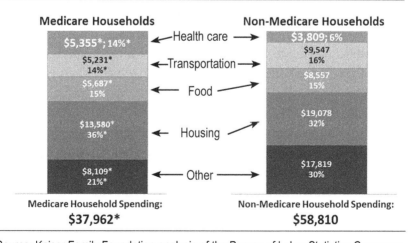

SHARE OF AVERAGE TOTAL HOUSEHOLD SPENDING ON HEALTH-RELATED EXPENSES
More than twice as large for Medicare households than for non-Medicare households in 2016

Source: Kaiser Family Foundation analysis of the Bureau of Labor Statistics Consumer Expenditure Survey Interview and Expense Files, 2016.

The safety net for seniors is further threatened by proposals from the GOP and Trump administration to cut Social Security as a way to reduce the federal deficit made worse by their own tax policies. Social Security already provides 90 percent of income for one-third of the elderly and a majority of cash income for 61 percent of seniors. [22]

4. Medicare Advantage gaming

Enrollment in private Medicare Advantage plans has doubled since 2010 to now cover 20 million U. S. seniors. They have been offering better benefits than public Medicare, and even promoted by Seema Verma, administrator of the Center for Medicare and Medicaid Services (CMS). There are a number of catches to these claims, however, as many enrollees find themselves later being dis-enrolled from Medicare Advantage plans and returning to original Medicare. It is true that many of these private plans offer benefits not available on public Medicare, such as vision and dental coverage. However, they commonly bait and switch with attractive premiums, then have other ways to game the system in favor of the plans and against the interests of their enrollees.

Medicare Advantage plans limit choice through restricted networks of physicians and hospitals, game reimbursement in their favor by up-coding of billable diagnoses, deny services to keep their costs down, dis-enroll sicker patients who diminish their profits and cost the government at least 14 percent more than public Medicare, even as they accept large annual overpayments from the government as "risk adjustment" payments. [23, 24]

5. Cutbacks in Medicaid

The Trump budget, as proposed but not yet implemented, would slash Medicaid, as the main safety net funding for those needing nursing home care, by $1.4 trillion over the coming decade. It's even worse than that, since proposed cuts would also be made for Medicare ($554 billion) and Social Security ($10 billion).[25] As if that isn't bad enough, nursing homes get such poor reimbursement for patients on Medicaid (just $200 a day compared to $500 a day on traditional Medicare for short-term stays or $430 a day for patients on a private Medicare managed care plan), profit-driven nursing homes frequently evict patients taking too much care.

6. Developing dementia

As our population ages, we will see the number of seniors in the U. S. with dementia continue to grow from today's number of 5 million. Its prevalence increases with age so that up to 40 percent of people reaching 85 years of age are likely to develop cognitive impairment through one or another type of dementia. [26] Because there still is no cure for dementia, these patients have a prolonged expensive course of irreversible cognitive decline typically requiring increasing levels of care that cost an estimated $200 billion a year, more than for cancer or heart disease. [27]

Early and moderate dementia can, in the best case, be managed at home, but it often ends up requiring institutional care, especially in a nursing home, as cognitive decline progresses. It is an ongoing challenge, however, throughout its course to assemble and retain caregivers, whether at home or in another setting. Moreover, it is an even bigger challenge to afford the increasing costs of care, as this patient's experience illustrates:

> *Dr. Leon Lederman received his Ph.D. in physics from Columbia University in 1951, did pioneering research in subatomic physics as a professor at the University of Chicago, and later won the Nobel Prize in Physics in 1988. Just before his 90th birthday, he was found to have dementia, for which his care exhausted his finances. He was forced to sell his Nobel Prize medal to set aside needed funds, which was done online to provide $765,000 before taxes. After being advised to settle in a peaceful place, he and his wife Ellen moved to Driggs, Idaho, where he died in a nursing home in 2018 at the age of 96. [28]*

7. Extended home care

Many, if not most of us, would like to stay at home as we age with advancing chronic illnesses and disabilities, with or without dementia. As patients and their families deal with the possibilities, they need to develop a plan that is caring, affordable, and flexible enough to evolve through changing circumstances. That plan, of course, depends on available family support, finances, and available options in the community.

This patient's story illustrates some of the severe challenges of needing LTC for dementia, incontinence, and disturbed sleep patterns when continued home care becomes very difficult.

> *Mrs. B, 82, lives on the first floor of a city apartment with her husband of 55 years, also 82. She cannot walk, and needs multiple helpers to get her up eight steps to her apartment. The waiting list for other accessible housing is longer than her predicted life span. She needs total care, is incontinent, and wears a diaper. She can't see or hear well, and cries out every night for her husband, frightened of what may happen to her. He gets little sleep and is exhausted from losing sleep. They desperately need a home health aide for night care. She has Medicaid, which covers a home health aid during the day, but not round-the-clock help at home. Neither Mrs. B and Mr. B want nursing home placement yet, but what will happen next and will they be able to afford long-term care at home, which costs even more than a nursing home?* [29]*

8. Extended nursing home/assisted living care

Many situations frequently arise during a fragile elder's stay in a nursing home or assisted living facility that present difficult decisions for the patient and family. This is one of them:

> *Mrs. H became weaker, unable to walk independently, and no longer able to dress, bathe, or use the toilet in an assisted living facility. With severe dementia, she spoke less, and had spells when she would stare into space without*

saying anything. After one of these episodes, she was sent to an E. R., where she was found to have heart block. A pacemaker was recommended, but her mother had had one and lived on for 12 years without any quality of life, so that her six children regretted approving it. In this new situation, her children (including her physician daughter) were mostly opposed to the procedure. Mrs. H at first accepted "whatever the doctor recommended," but then changed her mind, saying "I don't want a pacemaker. You doctors do too much stuff to old people." The pacemaker was cancelled, and with the family's support, she was shifted to hospice and comfort care where she was. She did not die of dementia, as her mother had with muteness and bed-bound immobility, but of heart disease. Had she lived longer, she would have died of dementia, which she never wanted. [30]

Conclusion

Having seen how expensive LTC is for patients and their families, it is time to move to the next chapter to discuss what we are getting for our money.

References

1. Martin, AB, Hartman, M, Washington, B et al. National health care spending in 2017: Growth slows to pre-recession rates; share of GDP stabilizes. *Health Affairs*, December 6, 2018.

2. Phelan, M. Why won't Congress vote on Bernie Sanders' bill? *Social Security Works*, August 5, 2017.

3. Year one of KHN's 'Bill of the Month': A kaleidoscope of financial challenges. *Kaiser Health News*, December 21, 2018.

4. Healthcare costs reach $6,348 for the average American, $28,348 for a hypothetical family of four. *Milliman Medical Index*, July 25, 2019.

5. Altman, D. The medical bill score. How the public judges health care. *Axios*, October 3, 2017.

6. Mathews, AW. New tactics on health costs. *Wall Street Journal*, December 4, 2018, R 10.

7.   Szabo, L. Health care industry spends $30B a year pushing its wares, from drugs to stem cell treatment. *Kaiser Health News*, January 8, 2019.

8.   Report details how skyrocketing prescription drug costs are harming the nation's seniors. *Common Dreams*, March 26, 2018.

9.   Gillers, H. Retiree health benefits cut. *Wall Street Journal*, May 2, 2019.

10. Ollstein, AM. 'It was not real insurance.' *Politico*, October 5, 2018.

11. Gillers, H. Bull market isn't helping pensions. *Wall Street Journal*, April 11, 2019: B 1.

12. Hellmann, J. Study: Americans using less health care, but paying more for it. *The Hill*, January 23, 2018.

13. Knight, V. In 10 years, half of middle-income elders won't be able to afford housing, medical care. *Kaiser Health News*, April 24, 2019.

14. Ibid # 2.

15. Span, P. Many Americans will need long-term care. Most won't be able to afford it. *New York Times*, May 10, 2019.

16. Gillers, H. As retiree health care bills mount, some states have a solution: stop paying. *Wall Street Journal*, May 1, 2019.

17. Cubanski, J, Neuman, T, Smith, K. Medicare beneficiaries' out-of-pocket health care spending as a share of income now and projections for the future. *Kaiser Family Foundation*, January 2018.

18. 10 essential facts about Medicare and prescription drug spending. *Kaiser Family Foundation*. November 10, 2017.

19. Orgera, K, Damico, A, Neuman, T. The financial burden of health care spending: Larger for Medicare households than for non-Medicare households. *Kaiser Family Foundation*, March 1, 2018.

20. Mannes, G. The pension crisis at Congress's door. *AARP Bulletin,* July/August 2019, p, 20.

21. Ibid # 20.

22. vanden Heuvel, K. Voters must catch on to Republicans' con on health care. *The Washington Post*, October 24, 2018.

23. Galewitz, P. Medicare Advantage riding high as new insurers flock to sell to seniors. *Kaiser Health News*, October 15, 2018.

24. Pear, R. Medicare Advantage found to improperly deny many claims. *New York Times*, October 13, 2018.

25. Tracy, J, Dewey, C, Goldstein, A et al. Trump wants to overhaul America's safety net with giant cuts to housing, food stamps, and health care. *The Washington Post*, February 12, 2018.

26. *2017 Alzheimer's Disease Facts and Figures*. Alzheimer's Association, 2017.

27. Hurd, MD et al. Monetary costs of dementia in the United States. *N Engl J Med* 368 (14): 1326-1334, 2013.
28. Johnson, G. A Nobel Prize-winning physicist sold his medal for $765,000 to pay medical bills. *New York Times*, October 4, 2018.
29. Powell, T. *Dementia Reimagined: Building a Life of Joy and Dignity from Beginning to End.* New York. *Penguin Random House*, 2019, pp. 162-164.
30. Ibid # 29, pp. 10-17.

CHAPTER 4

UNACCEPTABLE QUALITY OF LONG-TERM CARE

As we saw in the last chapter, the costs of U.S. health care have been increasing exponentially over the last 40 years, thereby making the costs of LTC more unaffordable for most people needing it. It is therefore important that we ask what we are getting for our money.

This chapter has two goals: (1) to briefly discuss deregulation as relates to health care under the Trump administration; and (2) to give examples of widespread unacceptable care and fraud regardless of setting with inadequate accountability.

Deregulation in Health Care under Trump Administration

Getting rid of supposedly useless regulations has been a theme of Trump's first two and a half years in office. Just ten days after his inauguration, he issued an executive order calling for government agencies to kill two rules for every one they propose. With an overt goal to "deconstruct the administrative state," this new policy was welcomed by many trade organizations and corporate lobbyists.[1] Soon thereafter, Trump put out another executive order titled "Ethical Commitments by Executive Branch Appointees," but that was just window dressing that lowered ethical standards within his Cabinet and administration. Six months later, 74 lobbyists were working in his administration, 49 of whom had previously lobbied on behalf of clients. [2] Beyond that, Trump has given many waivers of these "ethical standards" to many individuals without transparency. [3]

These are some other ways that the Trump administration has relaxed regulations as industry-friendly policies:

- Asking health care providers of all types for recommendations as to how to waive or roll back the requirements of federal fraud and abuse that prohibit kickbacks and other payments intended to influence care for people on Medicare or Medicaid. This naive goal was to invite health care providers to "work together to coordinate care, share cost reductions and profits in ways that would not otherwise be allowed." That announcement ignited a lobbying frenzy recommending ways to negate existing federal kickback and self-referral laws. [4]

- Although it is well known that the more than $30 billion a year that the medical-industrial complex spends each year on marketing its wares drives more testing, treatments, and health care costs, yet oversight of marketing and advertising is still inadequate. The Trump administration has made no efforts to ban direct-to-consumer advertising, as most advanced countries have done for years. [5]

- Although nearly one-third of drugs approved by the FDA from 2001 to 2010 were withdrawn from the market for safety reasons, after receiving accelerated approvals and being widely available to the public, the Trump administration is pushing for less regulation and faster approvals, as desired by the pharmaceutical industry. [6]

- In its March 2018 report *Twenty-Seven Years of Pharmaceutical Industry Criminal and Civil Penalties: 1991 Through 2017*, Public Citizen found that criminal penalties for pharmaceutical companies dropped by 88 percent in the 2016-2017 period compared to the 2012-2013 period. [7]

Widespread Unacceptable Care and Fraud in Long-Term Care

Home LTC

Although many people would prefer to die in their own homes, many factors are involved in making that possible, such as their functional status, chronic illnesses, availability of family and other caregivers, the patient's and family's finances, and the design of the home itself. (Appendix 1)

Given favorable answers to all these considerations, LTC at home may work out well, even for patients with early or moderate dementia. But that is not the case for those with advanced dementia, who need high levels of 24-7 care for such common problems as bowel and bladder incontinence, disrupted sleep-wake cycles, mobility problems, agitation, paranoia, and wandering.

Family members provide 75 to 80 percent of LTC at home but this becomes highly stressful sooner than later. [8] The work is hard, never ending, and is often not appreciated by the patients themselves. In many cases, it becomes necessary to bring in paid help called personal care assistants (PCAs). Some can be identified by word of mouth within the community, others through home health agencies.

As we saw in the first chapter, PCAs are a vulnerable group themselves, grossly underpaid, 89 percent women, most without health insurance or paid sick leave. Many are on Medicaid and need food stamps to help support their own families. Because of the hard, poorly paid work, turnover rates in many agencies are above 50 percent. [9] In view of our aging population and increasing prevalence of dementia, the Bureau of Labor Statistics has projected that the personal care assistant will be the fastest growing occupation in the country between 2012 and 2022. [10]

Caregiving by family members and PCAs is the essence of person-centered care affording patients an opportunity to age in place. With much of this care covered by Medicaid, it has become a booming industry with many for-profit home health agencies, unfortunately poorly regulated with fraud and abuse rampant.

Despite the obstacles, end-of-life care at home has been increasing since 1999 as hospital deaths decline, but most patients with advancing dementia still end up in a nursing home or long-term care facility. [11] That will be a big group far into the future, as shown in Figure 4.1.

FIGURE 4.1

PROJECTED NUMBER OF PEOPLE AGED 65 AND OLDER IN THE U.S. POPULATION WITH ALZHEIMER'S DISEASE, 2010-2050

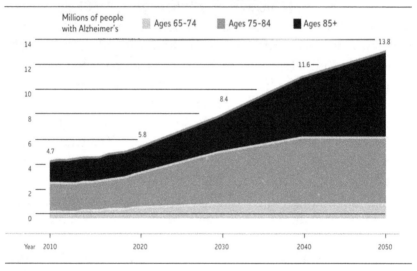

Source: Alzheimer's Association and National Institute on Aging of the National Institutes of Health

Assisted living

Assisted living facilities (ALFs) have grown rapidly over the last 25 years as a way for families to gain safe environments for their aging family members in a place that provides meals, housekeeping, 24-hour awake staff, transportation, and opportunities for social contact and activities. Most ALFs depend on private pay, some on a buy-in basis, while others may receive some Medicaid funding. They are intended as a bridge between home and nursing home. The biggest difference from nursing homes is the lack of 24-hour nursing care.

Although ALFs do not have skilled nursing care, they do provide help with activities of daily living (ADLs). According to a 2012 report of a national survey, more than one-third of assisted living residents receive assistance for three or more ADLs. (Figure 4.2) [12]

FIGURE 4.2

RESIDENTIAL CARE RESIDENTS RECEIVING ASSISTANCE WITH ACTIVITIES OF DAILY LIVING: U.S., 2010

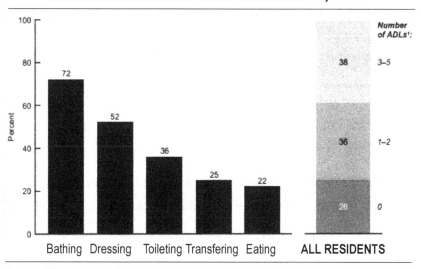

Source: CDC. National Center for Health Statistics, 2012

While there are many excellent assisted living places, they have become a growing, lucrative industry with almost no standards and little oversight by federal or state authorities. Residential assisted living has been hyped by private companies to Wall Street investors as "an explosive investment opportunity for the next 25 years." A 2018 report by the Government Accounting Office (GAO) found that only 22 states were able to furnish information on "critical incidents"—cases of potential or actual harm to patients. In one year, those states also reported a total of almost 23,000 such incidents involving physical, emotional, or sexual abuse of patients. [13]

Nursing homes

About two-thirds of the approximately 15,000 nursing homes in the U. S. are for profit, many of which in large chains. We know from many studies over past years that this is where the problems start. Compared to their not-for-profit counterparts, for-profit nursing homes have less RN nurse staffing despite sicker patients, worse quality of care and patient outcomes. The researchers observed the following strategies employed by the profit-hungry chains:

> *The chains have used strategies to maximize shareholder and investor value that include increasing Medicare revenues, occupancy rates, and company diversification, establishing multiple levels of corporate ownership, developing real estate trusts, and creating limited liability companies. These strategies enhance shareholder and investor profits, reduce corporate taxes, and reduce liability risk.* [14]

The worst abusers are the largest for-profit chains, such as HCR Manor Care, Golden Living, Life Care Centers of America, Kindred Healthcare, and Genesis HealthCare Corporation. [15] The Carlyle Group, one of the richest private-equity firms in the world, gives us one example of common abuse. After buying ManorCare, the second largest nursing home chain in the country, it announced hundreds of layoffs and staffing became inadequate, thereby leading to growing numbers of serious health code violations and harm to patients. After investors had extracted $1.3 billion from it, the company filed for bankruptcy. [16]

Here on our rural San Juan Island in Washington State, we had our own negative experience with Life Care Centers of America. It came in with its purchase of our long-standing, not-for-profit nursing home in 1997, making deep cuts in nursing staff and other costs, and then leaving abruptly at Thanksgiving time in 2017 with just three weeks' notice to patients and staff. One month earlier Life Care Centers of America announced that it had reached a settlement with the U. S. Department of Justice for $145 million (the largest in DOJ history) concerning allegations that it had charged for unnecessary treatments. [17] In its release, the DOJ stated that "Life Care submitted false claims for rehabilitation therapy by engaging in a systematic effort to increase its Medicare and TRI-CARE billings. . . Life Care also sought to keep patients longer than was necessary in order to continue billing for rehabilitation therapy, even after the treating therapists felt the therapy should be discontinued." [18]

There is another national scam involving U. S. nursing homes that has been uncovered through an analysis by *Kaiser Health News (KHN)* of federal inspection, staffing, and financial records for nursing homes across the country. It uncovered an increasingly common business arrangement whereby owners of nursing homes outsource a wide variety of goods and services to companies in which they have business dealings—a practice known as *related party transactions*. Owners can thereby enter into favorable contracts in which nursing homes pay more than they would have in a competitive market, then siphon off higher profits that are not recorded in their nursing home accounts. The KHN analysis documented that:

- Nursing homes that did business with sister companies employed, on average, 8 percent fewer nurses and aides.
- As a group, these homes were 9 percent more likely to have hurt residents or put them in immediate jeopardy of harm, and amassed 653 validated complaints for every 1,000 beds, compared with 32 per 1,000 that inspectors found credible at independent homes.
- Homes with related companies were fined 22 percent more often for serious health violations than were independent homes, and penalties averaged $24,441—7 percent higher. [19]

As if this is not bad enough, there are still other national scams involving nursing homes. Here is one more among others:

- Nursing homes, especially privately owned, often over sedate elderly residents with unneeded powerful psychotropic drugs in order to quiet them down, reduce their staffing needs, and gain more profits from Medicaid and Medicare reimbursement. [20] A statewide investigation by the *Chicago Tribune* of Illinois nursing homes found that this practice can lead to tremors, dangerous lethargy, a higher risk of falls, and even death. [21]

The Trump administration has aided and abetted this harmful, profiteering abandonment of the most vulnerable among us—patients in nursing homes. It has scaled back the use of fines against nursing homes that harm patients. [22] In addition, it imposed an 18-month moratorium in February 2018 on imposing fines or denials of federal payments when nursing homes fail to meet such requirements as ensuring that they have adequate staffing or are using psychotropic drugs correctly. [23]

Hospice

We might think that hospice, above all, might not be vulnerable to fraud and abuse, but we would be wrong. While hospice is intended to provide peaceful, comfort-oriented end of life care to patients in their last six months of life, with ready availability of caregivers, this is far from what happens in this booming industry which "served" about 1.4 million Medicare patients in 2015, one-third of Americans who died that year. [24]

A 2013 investigation by *The Washington Post* found that the number of for-profit hospices almost doubled from 2000 to 2013 while Medicare spending for hospice care increased five-fold. A common finding was that these hospice companies sought out less sick people who would require less care and live longer, thereby yielding higher profits. Some even paid kickbacks to referral sources, such as nursing homes, and offered bonuses to their employees to recruit such patients. [25,26]

A 2017 analysis by *Kaiser Health News* of some 20,000 government inspection records from the country's 4,000 plus hospice agencies revealed that missed visits and neglect are common for patients dying at home. More than 3,200 complaints had been filed with state officials over the past five years. One in five respondents said that their hospice did not show up in their time of need. Here is just one example, unfortunately not unusual, of this poor record:

> *Dr. Bob Martin, 66, retired family physician who had served his small, remote Alaska community for more than 30 years, had the misfortune to need urgent care over a long holiday weekend, when hospices are often too short-staffed to respond. With intense pain due to prostate cancer metastatic to his brain, his wife called many times for help. A nurse who was supposed to visit did not, and the supervising physician never responded. After six days and more calls, liquid methadone was finally received, but still no visit. He died just after midnight on January 4, 2014.* [27]

Medicaid fraud

Medicaid fraud and abuse is endemic in more than 30 states across the country, costing states billions of dollars each year and causing risk and potential harm to patients receiving unnecessary procedures. Private Medicaid plans are especially involved in fraud compared to their public counterparts, typically denying care through subcontractors owned by equity firms in order to maximize revenue for themselves and their shareholders. Unnecessary or duplicative payments to providers are common. [28, 29]

Fraud may take place at several levels:

- *by providers:* such as by billing for services not performed, duplicate billings, falsifying diagnoses, accepting kickbacks for patient referrals, ordering excessive or inappropriate tests, and/or prescribing medicines that are not medically necessary or for use by people other than the patient.
- *by insurers:* such as by misleading enrollees about health plan benefits, denying valid claims, overstating the insurer's cost in paying claims, and/or undervaluing the amount owed to health care providers.

- *by patients:* such as by providing false information to apply for services, using someone else's insurance coverage for services, filing claims for services or products not received, and/or obtaining medications or products that are not needed and selling them on the black market. [30]

Privatized Medicaid managed long-term care plans bring in further opportunities for fraud and abuse by insurers, including by cherry-picking healthy enrollees, falsifying enrollment information to obtain higher capitation rates, dis-enrolling expensive patients, denying medically necessary care, and contracting with unlicensed or unqualified providers. Leading insurers involved in these LTC plans that cover home and nursing home care under Medicaid include United Healthcare, Amerigroup, Centene, and Molina Healthcare. [31]

Here are two examples that illustrate the brazen magnitude of Medicaid fraud in opposite sides of the country:

- *The Money Laundering scheme during the tenure of Mitt Romney as governor of Massachusetts.* This was an elaborate operation involving illusory financing arrangements to claim federal Medicaid matching funds without actually spending the required state match. This is the same Romney who made the infamous "47 percent" comments against those who receive government assistance. [32, 33]
- *Questionable payments to California Medicaid managed care insurers.* California's Medicaid program, Medi-Cal, covers more than 13 million residents, one in three residents of the state. The State Auditor found "pervasive discrepancies" in Medicaid enrollment from 2014 to 2017 with some $3 billion being paid to insurers that contract with the state to provide managed care for 80 percent of enrollees in Medi-Cal. In one case, the state paid a managed care plan more than $380,000 to care for a person in Los Angeles County who had been dead for four years. [34]

Conclusion

What's in common here that ties this network of problems together and offers a way forward despite the greed of so many corporate stakeholders? Daniel Hatcher, Professor of Law at the University of Baltimore, examined the problems of the poverty industry in his 2016 book, *The Poverty Industry: The Exploitation of America's Most Vulnerable Citizens.* He drew this conclusion:

> *The poverty industry includes the vast combined powers of government and private enterprise. This collaboration has the capacity to do immense good, if the right goals are pursued.* [35]

References:

1. Steinzor, R. The war on regulation. *The American Prospect*, Spring 2017, pp. 72-76.
2. Nazaryan, A. The swamp runneth over. *Newsweek*, November 10, 2017.
3. Lipton, E, Ivory, D. Lobbyists, industry lawyers were granted ethics waivers to work in Trump administration. *New York Times*, June 8, 2017.
4. Pear, R. Trump administration invites health care industry to help rewrite ban on kickbacks. *New York Times*, November 24, 2018.
5. Szabo, L. Health care industry spends $30B a year pushing its wares, from drugs to stem cell treatment. *Kaiser Health News*, January 8, 2019.
6. Lupkin, S. Nearly 1 in 3 recent FDA drug approvals followed by major safety actions. *Kaiser Health News*, May 9, 2017.
7. Prupis, N. Penalties for PhRMA crimes have all but disappeared, report finds. *Public Citizen News*, May/June 2018, 11.
8. Spillman, B, Wolff, J, Freedman, V et al. *Informal caregiving for Older Americans: An Analysis of the 2011 National Health and Aging Trends Study.* Washington, D.C., U. S. Department of Health and Human Services.
9. *Paying the Price: How Poverty Wages Undermine Home Care in America*, Paraprofessional Healthcare Institute (PHI) February 16, 2015.
10. *Occupational projections for direct care workers*, Paraprofessional Healthcare Institute (PHI). 2014.
11. Hebert, LE, Weuve, PA, Scherr, DA et al. Alzheimer disease in the United States (2010 -2050) estimated using the 2010 census. *Neurology*, 2013.

12. CDC. National Center for Health Statistics, National Survey of Residential Care Facilities. Data Brief # 91, 2012.
13. Pear, R. U. S. pays billions for 'assisted living,' but what does it get? *New York Times*, February 3, 2018.
14. Harrington, C, Houser, C, Olney, B et al. Ownership, financing, and management strategies of the ten largest for-profit nursing home chains in the United States. *Intl. J Health Services* 41 (4):725-746, 2011.
15. Fernandez, E. Low staffing and poor quality of care at nation's for-profit nursing homes. *University of California San Francisco*, November 29, 2011.
16. Whoriskey, P, Keating, D. Overdoses, bedsores, broken bones: What happened when a private-equity firm sought to care for society's most vulnerable? *The Washington Post*, November 25, 2018.
17. Mongan, E. Feds finalize record $145 million settlement with Life Care Centers of America. *McKnights Long-Term Care News*, October 25, 2016.
18. Justice News. Life Care Centers of America Inc. agrees to pay $145 million to resolve False Claims Act allegations relating to provision of medically unnecessary rehabilitation therapy services. Washington, DC, *Department of Justice, Office of Public Affairs*, October 24, 2016.
19. Rau, J. Care suffers as more nursing homes feed money into corporate webs. *Kaiser Health News*, December 31, 2017.
20. Lagnado, L. Prescription abuse seen in U. S. nursing homes. *Wall Street Journal*, December 4, 2007.
21. Roe, S. Psychotropic drugs given to nursing home patients without cause. *Chicago Tribune*, October 27, 2009.
22. Weixel, N. Dems seek reversal of nursing home regulatory rollback. *The Hill*, February 20, 2018.
23. Gorman, A. Weak oversight blamed for poor care at California nursing homes going unchecked. *Kaiser Health News*, May 4, 2018.
24. Aleccia, JN, Bailey, M. No one is coming: Hospice patients abandoned at death's door. *Kaiser Health News*, October 26, 2017.
25. Hatcher, D. *The Poverty Industry: The Exploitation of America's Most Vulnerable Citizens.* New York. *New York University Press,* 2016, p. 205.
26. Paquette, D. End-of-life care: An industry with soaring profits, funded by taxpayers. *The Washington Post*, August 21, 2014.
27. Waldman, P. Preparing Americans for death lets hospices neglect end of life. *Bloomberg*, July 22, 2011.
28. Herman, B. Medicaid's unmanaged managed care. *Modern Healthcare*, April 30, 2016.
29. Bailey, M. Seniors suffer amid widespread fraud by Medicaid caretakers. *Kaiser Health News*, November 7, 2016.
30. Terhune, C. Coverage denied: Medicaid patients suffer as layers of private companies profit. *Kaiser Health News*, January 3, 2019.

31. Sheehan, JG. Fraud and abuse in managed long-term care. White paper, 2015. sheehanj@hra.nyc.gov
32. Ibid # 31.
33. Medicaid money laundering. *Wall Street Journal*, May 19, 2008.
34. Terhune, C. Billions in 'questionable payments' went to California's insurers and providers. *Kaiser Health News*, November 1, 2018.
35. Ibid # 25, p. 221.

PART II

HOW DID WE GET HERE?

CHAPTER 5

HISTORICAL PERSPECTIVE

Having looked in Part I at the major problems affecting LTC in the U. S., it is now useful to look back through history as to what brought us here. That will be necessary if we are to have any success in solving these problems, as we will discuss in Part III of this book.

For now, this chapter will sort through some of the major historical trends that underlie the challenges of providing long-term care in this country.

Historical Trends
1. Underestimating the increasing need for long-term care.

We still lack an organized system for providing long-term care. At least 90 percent of older people needing help with activities of daily living (ADLs) depend on "informal" care by family and friends, who collectively provide 75-80 percent of total care hours in non-institutional settings. [1] Older people needing LTC without such informal resources typically end up in nursing homes.

As we saw in Chapter 1, these are some of the ways that the need for LTC has been increasing over many years:

- Aging of our population (Figure 1.1, p.6).
- Six threats that collectively or separately threaten the capability of aging adults to cope with their changing circumstances (Table 1.1, p.8).
- Increased inequality.

- Increased disparities.
- Increased unaffordability of LTC with decline of long-term care insurance.
- Threats to Medicaid and the safety net.
- Threats to Social Security, which provides 90 percent of income for one-third of seniors and is under constant attack by Republicans who see its cuts as a way to reduce the federal deficit. [2]

Here are some additional ways that further exacerbate the growing crisis in LTC in this country:

- Continued reduction of defined benefit retirement plans as they are replaced by defined contribution plans, such as 401(k) plans. [3]
- Living beyond personal and family savings as inflation rates exceed cost of living.
- The projected increases in the number of people with Alzheimer's disease. (Figure 4.1, p. 52)
- Seniors are expected to outnumber children in the U. S. population by 2035. [4]
- The 80-plus part of the U. S. population will more than triple from 11 million in 2010 to 35 million in 2050. [5]
- The number of centenarians, those living to 100 or older, is projected by the Census Bureau to continue growing rapidly. (Figure 5.1) [6]
- Decreased marriage and birth rates of millennial generation (those born between 1981 and 1996), together with lower household net worth. [7]
- Shortage of caregivers is a risk to LTC. (Figure 5.2) [8]

FIGURE 5.1

ADULTS LIVING TO 100 YEARS OR OLDER IN THE U.S., 1980-2030

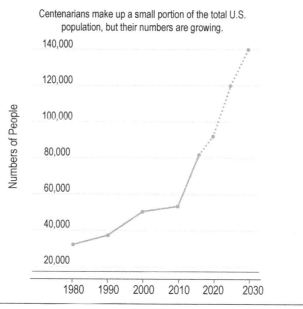

Centenarians make up a small portion of the total U.S. population, but their numbers are growing.

Source: Ansberry, C. The advantages and limitations of living to 100. *Wall Street Journal*, May 21, 2019.

FIGURE 5.2

CAREGIVER SUPPORT RATIO, 1980 TO 2050

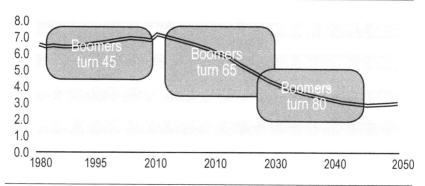

Note: The caregiver support ratio is the ratio of the population aged 45-64 to the population age 80-plus.
Source: AARP Report. *The Aging of the Baby Boom and the Growing Care Gap: A Look at Future Declines in the Availability of Family Caregivers.*

2. Under recognizing our country's cultural disrespect for aging, disabilities, and dementias over many years

Dr. Tia Powell, whom we met in Chapter 1, brings this insight to how we have seen dementia, as one example of people needing LTC over the years, with important implications of how unadvanced we are in our societal response to those needing such care.

The history of our cultural response to dementia is not pretty. Looking back over the centuries, we find those with dementia in jail, in workhouses, in shackles, and in mental institutions. We have punished rather than treated. We have shown those who need help that they are a nuisance, a bother. The help that was offered in centuries past was designed to chastise, control, and minimize the trouble for minders while the inmates waited for death. Even today, we find those with dementia in our jails and homeless shelters. The way a society treats people with dementia creates a portrait of that society. In looking at how we respond to them, we see ourselves. [9]

Here are some nodal points along the way since the 1800s:

- In the 1800s, there was no safety net as poor people were pushed into poorhouses or jails together with the unemployed and people with physical and mental disabilities. [10]
- Early 1800s—first mental hospitals established as asylums for the mentally ill; patients were often in restraints.
- The number of public mental institutions doubled between 1870 and 1890, each often housing 800 to 1,000 patients. [11]
- Early 1900s—first reports of what became known as Alzheimer's disease.
- 1920s through 1960s—hospitalized psychiatric patients faced invasive experimental treatments, such as lobotomy and electroconvulsive therapy (ECT), often without the right to refuse.

- 1946—Congress created the National Institute of Mental Health (NIMH) for funding of research on psychiatric illness.
- 1960s—start of closures of state mental hospitals, shifting mainly to nursing homes for custodial care of isolated poor elderly, many with dementia.
- 1965—passage of Medicare and Medicaid; Medicare covered short stays regardless of income, while Medicaid covered long-term care for low income patients.
- 1993—Tacrine was approved as first of many drugs to follow for Alzheimer's disease, none of which have been curative.
- 1999—Olmstead decision by the U. S. Supreme Court, finding that disabled persons had the right to receive care in the least possible restrictive setting; that led to deinstitutionalization of mental health care and the growth of other community-based facilities.
- 2010—passage of the Affordable Care Act without a provision sponsored by Senator Ted Kennedy, the Community Living Assistance Services and Supports Act (CLASS Act) that was intended to help pay for the costs of LTC. [12]

3. Changing locations for long-term care

Sweeping changes have taken place over the last two-plus centuries in America that reflect changing societal structure. Most LTC was provided in the home in earlier years, when families were larger, family members less mobile and more attuned to care for their elders. Then came the big shift to state mental hospitals for those with dementias or other frailties, which then went to nursing homes when the mental hospitals were largely shut down. More recently, as we have seen, is the further shift to assisted living facilities, other community-based options, and hospices for those in their last six months of life.

What was possible and common 100 years ago seems idyllic today—staying in one's own home, with younger family caregivers still in the community and willing to devote much of their lives to care of their aging and increasingly frail parents and grandparents. Most Americans still want to age in place in their own homes, but that has become increasingly impossible, given smaller families, greater mobility of younger family members fully involved in their own lives, unaffordable costs of other caregivers if they are even available, and high costs of other locations, such as nursing homes and assisted living facilities.

4. For-profit privatization leading to increasing unaffordability of long-term care

In his farewell address in 1961, President Dwight Eisenhower warned of a military-industrial complex of defense contracting whereby funds intended to serve the public would be diverted to benefit the self-interest of government actors and private contractors. As he said at the time:

> *The potential for disastrous rise of misplaced power exists and will persist.* [13]

That warning, of course, went unheeded as the trend toward privatization across our economy grew rapidly, based on the discredited myth that the private sector can perform better than government. Two decades later, Dr. Arnold Relman, internist and former editor of *The New England Journal of Medicine*, gave us this similar warning for health care:

> *The new "medical-industrial complex" may be more efficient than its not-for-profit competition, but it creates the problems of overuse and fragmentation of services, overemphasis on technology, and "cream skimming", and it may also exercise undue influence on national health policy. Closer attention from the public and the profession, and careful study are necessary to ensure that the "medical-industrial complex" puts the interests of the public before those of its stockholders.* [14]

Again, this warning went unheeded as the inevitable wave of privatization engulfed U. S. health care, and converted much of it to corporate for-profit enterprises beholden more to CEOs, Wall Street, and shareholders than to the needs of patients and their families. The Congressional Research Service, the research division of the Library of Congress, urged caution about privatization by the federal government in these words: "contracting out can promote iron triangles and other corrupt relationships between the federal government and the private sector." [15]

Long-term care has become just another target for government enabled-private sector profiteering best described as "poverty's iron triangle" by Professor Daniel Hatcher in his 2016 book, *The Poverty Industry: The Exploitation of America's Most Vulnerable Citizens.* This iron triangle involves both state and federal government with self-serving interests and conflicts of interest that adversely impact children, seniors, and the most vulnerable among us.

One example, among many described by Professor Hatcher, is a scheme that was developed in Indiana where the largest public hospital system bought up for-profit nursing homes, used them to increase federal Medicaid payments, then diverted those funds for purposes other than improving care for residents of the nursing homes. [16] Figure 5.3 shows how these inter-relationships work. [17]

Did the passage of the Affordable Care Act (ACA) in 2010 do anything to rein in these blatant attacks on the public interest? No way, as Theodore Marmor, professor emeritus of public policy and management at Yale University, and his colleagues summarized in their 2014 book, *Social Insurance: America's Neglected Heritage and Contested Future*:

Little if anything in the ACA addresses the fundamental causes of the rampant inflation in medical care that has consumed greater portions of Americans' income over past decades. Medical inflation will likely continue to plague public, personal, and corporate budgets. . . Despite virtually no evidence of cost-control success, the plea to let market competition work its wonders will remain a refrain of American medical care debates. [18]

FIGURE 5.3

POVERTY'S IRON TRIANGLE

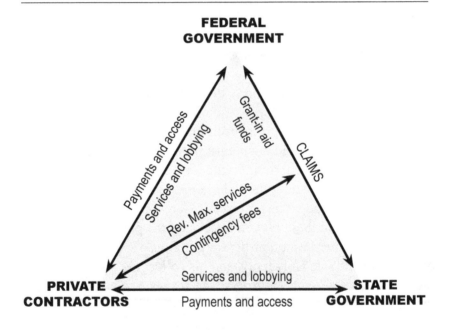

Source: Hatcher D.L., *The Poverty Industry: The Exploitation of America's Most Vulnerable Citizens*

5. *Lack of a national policy and continuing neglect of the problem*

The foregoing makes clear that we have failed to develop any kind of a rational plan to deal with the increasing stakes of LTC in this country. Even as the need for more LTC has grown exponentially for many decades, we still haven't even approached the task of formulating a national plan. We just drift along while corporate interests steal the day and increasingly draw down public and private budgets in their own self-interest.

Dr. Henry Moss, Ph.D. (in philosophy) is author of the excellent 2015 book, *The 2030 Caregiving Crisis: A Heavy Burden for Boomer Children*. A retired baby boomer himself, he has written on cognitive science and the history and philosophy of technological progress. His interests range from health care to housing and urban development to theories of social development. With Medicare funding, he calls for the training of millions of personal care aides as respected paraprofessionals, together with their higher compensation, improved training and working conditions. We will include his other recommendations in Chapter 11. [19]

Conclusion

We will return to future planning for LTC in the last three chapters of Part III, but for now, let's turn to one of the biggest culprits guarding the unacceptable status quo—privatization and failure of our vaunted competitive markets.

References

1. Spillman, B, Wolff, J, Freedman, V et al. *Informal Caregiving for Older Americans: An Analysis of the 2011 National Health and Aging Trends Study*. U. S. Department of Health and Human Services, Washington, DC, 2014.
2. vanden Heuvel, K. Voters must catch on to Republicans' con on health care. *The Washington Post*, October 24, 2018.

3. Pension Benefit Guaranty Corporation, 2011 PBGC Annual Report, Washington, DC

4. Anderson, S. America needs a long-term care program for seniors. *Common Dreams*, May 22, 2019.

5. Redfoot, D, Feinberg, L, Houser, A. The aging of the baby boom and the growing care gap: A look at future declines in the availability of family caregivers. (Insight on the Issues Report 85). Washington, DC *AARP Public Policy Institute.*

6. Ansberry, C. The advantages and limitations of living to 100. *Wall Street Journal*, May 21, 2019.

7. Adamy, J, Overberg, P. Millennials near middle age in crisis. *Wall Street Journal*, May 20, 2019: A1.

8. Moss, M. *The 2030 Caregiving Crisis: A Heavy Burden for Boomer Children*. Bronx, N. Y. *Henry Moss,* 2015, pp. 3-7.

9. Powell, T. *Dementia Reimagined: Building a Life of Joy and Dignity from Beginning to End*. New York. *Penguin Random House*, 2019, p. 21.

10. Ibid # 28, p. 29.

11. Grob, GN. *Mental Illness and American Society,* 1875-1940. Princeton, N.J. *Princeton University Press*, 1987, p. 76.

12. Gleckman, H. Requiem for the CLASS Act. *Health Affairs* 30 (12), 2011, 2231-2234.

13. President Dwight D. Eisenhower, Farewell Address, January 17, 1961.

14. Relman, AS. The new medical-industrial complex. *N Engl J Med* 303: 963-970, 1980.

15. Kosar, KR. Congressional Research Service. *Privatization and the Federal Government: An Introduction*, December 28, 2006.

16. Hatcher DL, *The Poverty Industry: The Exploitation of America's Most Vulnerable Citizens*. New York. *New York University Press*, 2016, p.55.

17. Ibid # 16, p. 5.

18. Marmor, TR, Mashaw, J, Pakutka, J. *Social Insurance: America's Neglected Heritage and Contested Future*. Washington, DC, *Sage COPRESS*, 2014, p. 126.

19. Ibid # 8. p. 10.

CHAPTER 6

MARKET FAILURE
AND PRIVATIZATION

This chapter has two goals: (1) to discuss the history, track record, and failure of market-based strategies for U. S. health care; and (2) to describe the growing role of privatization that results in decreased access to more unaffordable and worse health care for patients and their families.

Ongoing Market Failure

Most economists since the 1960s have believed that an unfettered competitive marketplace can resolve system problems of access, cost and quality in U. S. health care. This myth has been around so long as to become a meme, and even the "American way." Few economists have questioned this belief, despite incontrovertible evidence over the last 50 years that health care markets do not behave in a freely competitive way.

As we saw in the last chapter, Dr. Arnold Relman's warning about the downsides of a medical-industrial complex have gone unheeded since 1980. The same is true about the issue of how markets work in health care. We should have listened to these prescient warnings by two economists before their time:

- Dr. Kenneth Arrow, a leading economist at Columbia University, predicted as early as 1963 that uncertainty would be the root cause of market failure in health care, both for patients and physicians dealing with unavoidable uncertainties concerning diagnosis, treatment, and prognosis of illness. [1]
- Joseph Stiglitz, Ph.D., Nobel Laureate in Economics and former chief economist at the World Bank, had this to say in 2004:

Markets do not lead to efficient outcomes, let alone outcomes that comport with social justice. As a result, there is often good reason for government intervention to improve the efficiency of the market. Just as the Great Depression should have made it evident that the market does not work as well as its advocates claim, our recent Roaring Nineties should have made it self-evident that the pursuit of self-interest does not necessarily lead to overall economic efficiency. [2]

There are many reasons why markets do not work in health care as they do in other areas, such as buying a car. One reason is the asymmetry of information on the part of patients vs. providers promoting their products or services to patients. Prices of health care services are not readily available to the public, so that most patients do not know the eventual costs of the care they agree to. As a result, it is difficult or impossible to shop around for care, especially given the frequent problem of urgency of time. Another big reason is that profit incentives among providers of care work against the goals of patients to gain access to care at the lowest and most affordable cost. As Robert Evans, Ph.D., health care economist at the University of British Columbia noted more than 20 years ago, market mechanisms in health care yield distributional advantages to different groups, including a natural alliance among providers, suppliers, and insurers to increase their profits as they sell their services to patients. [3]

The increasing consolidation of giant corporations through mergers makes it even more difficult for patients to gain access to affordable care. As they acquire increasing market share, these large corporations have wide latitude to set prices that disadvantage patients even more. In our current industry-friendly deregulated market, power in the marketplace increasingly favors the interests of corporate stakeholders vs. the needs of patients as corporate giants cross over to other areas of health care. Two good examples of this growing trend are the acquisition of large physician groups by UnitedHealth Group, the largest private insurer in the country,[4] and the recent purchase of Aetna, the third largest insurer, by CVS Health, which has some 10,000 pharmacy and clinic locations around the country. [5]

Here are just two examples of how patients are disadvantaged in trying to find affordable care:

> *Benjamin Hynden, a financial advisor in Fort Meyers, Florida, saw his physician after not feeling well with discomfort in his abdomen for several weeks. No treatment was recommended at the time after examination, evaluation, and a normal CT scan. His bill was $268 for these services. Three months later, he still didn't feel well and tried to see the same physician, who was not available. He saw a nurse practitioner, who advised him to go to an ER, where a triage nurse said that the problem was not his appendix, but still recommended another CT scan. That was done, by the very same machine, with a normal result, and he was again sent home without a definitive diagnosis. The bill for the second CT scan of the abdomen was $8,897, more than 33 times the bill for the first CT scan!* [6]

> *Kim Daniels had full coverage by her insurer, PennCare, when she had a double mastectomy and reconstructive surgery for breast cancer in June, 2018. Because of that coverage, cost didn't seem to be an issue in selecting what kind of breast implant to choose. She decided upon high-end Mentor MemoryGel implants costing $3,500 each, $7,000 for the pair, all covered by insurance. It turns out, however, that this price is much higher with the insurer paying for the implants than it would have been had Kim received them for cosmetic breast augmentation, which is generally not covered by insurance. In that case, that same $7,000 would have covered the doctors' fees, anesthesia, and operating room time, as well as the implants that cost the providers a maximum of $3,000 for a set. This big difference is due to who is paying—if patients were paying, as for cosmetic surgery, providers have to offer the implants close to their own costs in order to compete with other cosmetic surgeons.* [7]

The Increasing Privatization of U. S. Health Care

Although privatization was not in our vernacular 60 years ago, it has become a driving force throughout our economy ranging from schools, water and the military to health care. Its early history in health care is especially interesting. When Lyndon Johnson became president in 1964, Democrats controlled both chambers in Congress, including a two to one majority in the House. Despite the strong opposition by the American Medical Association, Medicare was enacted in July 1965 as a "three-layer cake" that put together three different proposals—Medicare Part A (universal hospital coverage for the elderly), Medicare Part B (voluntary, supplemental physician coverage for the elderly), and Medicaid (an expansion of the Kerr-Mills federal-state program for indigent health care).

In what later became known as the "corporate compromise of 1965," this combination was intended to limit further expansion of social insurance (such as Medicare Part A, universal and not-for-profit) and open new private markets in health care. (It was passed by overwhelming majorities in Congress—by votes of 307 to 116 in the House and by 70 to 24 in the Senate). [8]

Private insurers were relieved of their worse health risks, the elderly and the poor, as they focused on younger, healthier, lower-risk enrollees. They gained even more as the day-to-day administration of the program was contracted out to private providers and intermediaries, including Blue Cross, for claims processing, provider reimbursement, and auditing. Hospitals won by getting generous reimbursement for a previously disadvantaged population. Physicians became compensated for the care of many lower-income patients for whom they previously had rendered care on a charity basis. [9,10]

Privatization of government health programs gained momentum during the Nixon administration in 1972, when Social Security amendments were enacted authorizing Medicare to contract with private health maintenance organizations (HMOs). Ten years later, Congress passed the Tax Equity and Fiscal Responsibility

Act of 1982, by which Medicare could pay HMOs 95 percent of what traditional Medicare would pay for fee-for-service care in beneficiaries' county of residence. That number was based on the supposed greater efficiency of the private sector, but soon launched a gaming system whereby private HMOs gamed the system for much higher overpayments reaching some $283 billion between 1985 and 2008.[11] These overpayments continue today without any constraints.

Conservative politicians and policy makers have continuously pressed for more privatization of health care as it became redefined as a commodity to be bought and sold on private markets. In its quest for smaller government and supposed fiscal austerity, the GOP has long wanted to constrain and even kill Medicare. Newt Gingrich, as Speaker of the House in a new Republican-controlled Congress in 1995, brought a bill forward to privatize Medicare (later vetoed by President Clinton), saying that this kind of "reform" might "solve the Medicare problem and lead to its withering on the vine." [12]

That approach by conservatives has continued to this day despite the long track record of privatized programs being less efficient than their public counterparts, being more expensive, restricting access, and providing worse care.

Instead of better results through private programs, we have seen the growth of a large corporate welfare system that continues to feed on public programs at the expense of patients, families and taxpayers. Ralph Nader, longtime consumer advocate, attorney, and co-founder of Public Citizen, has observed:

> *Big corporations should not be allowed the myths of competitive, productive, efficient capitalism—unless they can prove it.* [13]

Unfortunately, the service ethic has lost out to the supposed business "ethic" as profit-oriented privatization continues across the health care system. Figure 6.1 shows how widely it had spread throughout our market-based "system" by 2016, more than many people realize. Any part of privatized health care has come to mean higher prices, less service, more bureaucracy, profiteering, and often corruption as private companies and contractors keep dipping into the public till at taxpayer expense.

FIGURE 6.1

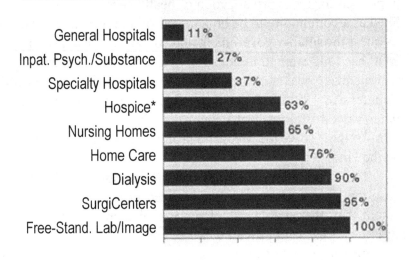

EXTENT OF FOR-PROFIT OWNERSHIP 2016

Source: Commerce Dept. *Service Annual Surveys and MedPac*, Data are Q1, 2016 or most recent available.

Here is what the territory looks like today as we view the U. S. health care system in 2020.

Medicare

The Trump administration has been blatantly promoting Medicare Advantage (or Medicare Disadvantage more accurately!) as if private is better than the original public Medicare program. Subject lines in emails from the administration to millions of beneficiaries have extolled the virtues of private Medicare plans in such words as "get more benefits for your money," "with Medicare Advantage, one plan covers all of your care," and "see if you can save money with Medicare Advantage." Richard F. Foster, former nonpartisan chief actuary of the Medicare program, called these emails "more like Medicare Advantage plan advertising than objective information from a public agency." [14].

While Medicare Advantage can offer a few services not covered by traditional Medicare (such as vision, hearing, and dental care), it does so by deceptive marketing methods. In promising predictable costs and extra value through "choice and competition," the Trump administration is weaving a tangle of lies and disinformation, avoiding mention of these kinds of problems:

- Private Medicare Advantage plans gravitate to markets without competition; a 2015 report by the Commonwealth Fund found that 97 percent of markets for these plans were "highly concentrated" with little competition.[15]
- Private insurers often hold marketing meetings in upstairs buildings without elevators in order to select out healthier enrollees from sicker ones.
- All possible diagnoses are used to up-code billings, often gained through retrospective chart reviews, but unrelated to services that patients actually received. [16]
- Limited choice of physicians and hospitals through restricted networks.
- Frequent denial of claims. [17]
- Frequent disenrollment if enrollees get sick and start costing insurers too much.
- The Trump administration now allows private insurers to charge seniors five times as much as younger people for premiums, compared to a 3:1 ratio enacted under the ACA. [18]
- Administrative costs 5 times higher than Medicare's 2.5 percent.
- High federal overpayments for many years, including at least $30 billion in the last three years alone. [19] (Figure 6.2)

FIGURE 6.2

MEDICARE OVERPAYS PRIVATE PLANS

Total Overpayments 2008-2016: $173.7 billion

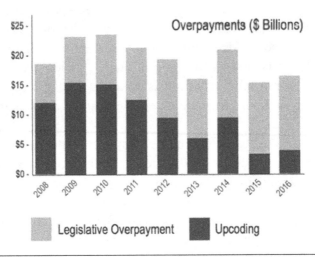

Source: Schulte, F, Weber, L. Medicare Advantage overbills taxpayers by billions a year as feds struggle to stop it. *Kaiser Health News*, July 16, 2019.

What privatized Medicare plans actually do, after a long track record over many years, is summarized in Table 6.1 comparing public and private Medicare.

Medicaid

Privatized Medicaid follows the same pattern as privatized Medicare, with poor service, inadequate physician networks, long waits for care, and denials of many treatments, even as the insurers take in new profits. Centene Corp., the largest Medicaid insurer in the country, raked in $1.1 billion in profits between 2014 and 2016, even as its plans were among the worst performing in California. [20] Private managed care plans frequently game the system for increased profits by falsifying records, colluding bid-rigging, and withholding payments to providers or subcontractors. Overpayments to these plans are common in more than 30 states, often involving duplicative payments to providers and calling for more scrutiny by auditors. [21]

TABLE 6.1

COMPARATIVE FEATURES OF PRIVATIZED AND PUBLIC MEDICARE

PRIVATIZED MEDICARE	ORIGINAL MEDICARE
Experience-rated eligibility	Universal coverage
Managed competition	Social insurance as earned right
Defined contribution	Defined benefits
Segmented risk pool	Broad risk pool
Market pricing to risk	Administered prices
More volatile access & benefits	More reliable access & benefits
Increased cost sharing	Less cost sharing
Less accountability	Potential for more accountability
Less choice of provider & hospital	Full choice of provider & hospital
Less well distributed	Well distributed
Less efficiency, higher overhead	More efficiency, lower overhead

Source: Geyman, J. *Shredding the Social Contract, The Privatization of Medicare*, Monroe, ME. *Common Courage Press*, 2006, p. 206

Private insurers

Since the ACA was enacted in 2010, private insurers became involved with the exchanges in many new ways, including determining eligibility for qualified health plans and subsidies/tax credits, as well as verifying annual household income and family size. Since income usually varies from year to year, this brought increasing bureaucracy and administrative revenue. Insurers have been gaming the ACA's risk-coding program, which rewards them more by covering older and sicker enrollees, by overstating their health risks. [22] The bureaucracy of private insurers has further increased over the last two years as the Trump administration experiments with work requirements in some state Medicaid programs, thereby requiring ongoing monitoring of who is working, and changing often in hourly or temporary jobs. [23]

Profit margins of several top insurers for the first quarter of 2018 were the highest in a decade. CEOs of the six largest insurers took in more that $17 million each in 2017. [24] A national study by Covered California projects that cumulative premium increases by private insurers for 2019 to 2021 will range from 35 percent to more than 90 percent. [25]

Hospitals

In this age of increasing consolidation among large corporate mergers, it is well documented that expanding hospital systems, facing less competition and gaining market power, charge much higher prices, even by up to 40 to 50 percent. [26] Prices vary widely, even within the same state. As one example among many, hospital charges for a routine appendectomy in California have been found to range from $1,500 to $182,955! [27]

Doctor-owned hospitals are a special problem that flies under the radar. They focus on well-reimbursed services and procedures, such as in cardiovascular disease and orthopedic surgery, as a way for physicians to evade laws prohibiting them from referring patients to hospitals in which they are invested. They typically cherry pick well insured patients, then charge patients higher bills by "triple dipping" as their physician owners profit by receiving income from performing a procedure, sharing in a facility profit, and increasing the value of their investment in the business. [28]

Nursing homes

A number of examples of the drive toward revenue generation rather than service to patients were mentioned earlier in Chapters 2 and 4. As we saw, many nursing homes across the country have dangerously low staffing levels, unacceptable quality of care, and evict patients when they are no longer profitable. Investor-owned nursing home chains often engage poor care practices and conceal bad outcomes while having higher rates of patient injury than their not-for-profit counterparts. [29] A recent study involving 55,000 patients in more than 600 nursing homes in New York State found

that physical, occupational and speech therapy were being continued into the last 30 days of life for 7,600 patients when palliative
care and hospice were indicated. [30] Despite these glaring and continuing problems, regulatory oversight remains weak. In response,
Illinois has just passed a bill requiring nursing home violators to
advertise any state staffing violations on their websites, in their
main lobbies, at their registration desks, and at every public entry-
way to the facility. [31]

Home care

The profit motive even extends into home care, with three
of four home health agencies across the country being for-profit.
They have been documented to have higher costs and lower quality of care than their not-for-profit counterparts. [32]

Emergency medical services

In the aftermath of the 2008-2009 recession, many cities and
towns across the country struggled to afford ambulance services.
Private equity came to the "rescue" with a mission to make as
much money as possible from this public need. A 2016 report from
the *New York Times* exposed practices that often endangered the
lives of patients, such as ambulances with expired medications and
delayed response times even to the point of non-availability. Cost
cutting, price increases, and aggressive billing practices were all
part of the picture. [33]

Conclusion

With privatized, often corporatized health care programs, the
story is always the same private profits, no price controls, less
affordable, less choice, worse care, more profiteering, and inadequate accountability. They increase patient and family debt, lead
to more borrowing, and often result in personal bankruptcies, two-
thirds of which in the U. S. are caused by illness and medical bills.
This situation endangers the lives of our fellow Americans, vio-
lates the public trust, and is unsustainable. Can't we do better?

Lawrence Brown, professor of public policy and management at Columbia University, brings us this important insight about the downsides of privatized health care:

> *No other nation expects a private sector, little constrained by public rules on the size and terms of employer contributions, to carry so heavy a burden of coverage and none asks private insurers to hold the line with providers (including specialists, uncommonly abundant in the United States) on prices outside a framework of public policies that guide the bargaining game. The first of these two grand exceptions largely accounts for the nation's high rates of un- and underinsurance; the latter mainly explains why America's health spending is so high by cross-national standards.*[34]

This observation leads us to the next chapter, where we will consider how the lack of adequate insurance stands as a barrier to long-term care that most of us will eventually need.

References

1. Arrow, K. Uncertainty and the welfare economics of medical care. *American Economic Review* 53: 941-973, 1963.
2. Stiglitz, JE. Evaluating economic change. *Daedalus* 133/3, Summer, 2004.
3. Evans, RG, Going for the gold: The redistributive agenda behind market-based health care reform. *J Health Polit. Policy Law* 22: 427-465, 1997.
4. Abelson, R. UnitedHealth buys large doctors group as lines blur in health care. *New York Times*, December 6, 2017.
5. de la Merced, MJ, Abelson, R. CVS to buy Aetna for $69 billion in a deal that may reshape the health industry. *New York Times*, December 3, 2017.
6. Kodjak, A. A tale of two CT scanners—one richer, one poorer. *Kaiser Health News*, April 9, 2018.
7. Knight, V. One implant, two prices. It depends on who's paying. *Kaiser Health News*, December 11, 2018.
8. Marmor, TR. *The Politics of Medicare*. Second edition, New York. *Aldine de Gruyter*, 2000, pp. 45-57.

9. Gordon, C. *Dead on Arrival: The Politics of Health Care in Twentieth Century America*. Princeton, NJ. *Princeton University Press*, 2003, pp. 25-28.
10. Oberlander, J. *The Political Life of Medicare*. Chicago. *The University of Chicago Press*, 2003, pp. 108-112.
11. Trivedi, AN, Gribla, R, Jiang, L et al. Duplicate federal payments to dual enrollees in Medicare Advantage programs and the Veterans Affairs Health Care System. *JAMA* 308 (1):67-72, 2012.
12. Hacker, JS. *The Divided Welfare State: The Battle Over Public and Private Social Benefits in the United States*. Cambridge. *Cambridge University Press*, 2002, p. 329.
13. Nader, R. The myths of big corporate capitalism. In the Public Interest. *The Progressive Populist*, August 15, 2015, p. 19.
14. Foster, RS, as quoted by Pear, R. Trump administration peppers inboxes with plugs for private Medicare plans. *New York Times*, December 1, 2018.
15. Abelson, R. With mergers, concerns grow about private Medicare. *New York Times*, August 25, 2015.
16 Geruso, M, Layton, T. Up-coding inflates Medicare costs in excess of $2 billion annually. *UT News, University of Texas at Austin*, June 18, 2015.
17. Pear, R. Medicare Advantage found to improperly deny many claims. *New York Times*, October 13, 2018.
18. Richtman, M. GOP's proposed Medicare voucher program would lead to demise of the system. *The Hill*, March 5, 2018.
19. Schulte, F, Weber, L. Medicare Advantage overbills taxpayers by billions a year as feds struggle to stop it. *Kaiser Health News*, July 16, 2019.
20. Terhune, C, Gorman, A. Enriched by the poor: California health insurers make billions through Medicaid. *Kaiser Health News*, November 6, 2017.
21. Herman, B. Medicaid's unmanaged managed care. *Modern Healthcare*, April 30, 2016.
22. Potter, W. Health insurers working the system to pad their profits. *Center for Public Integrity*, August 15, 2015.
23. Corcoran, M. Medicaid work requirements: Trump's war on the poor expands, one state at a time. *Truthout*, April 25, 2018.
24. The high cost of healthcare: Patients see greater cost-shifting and reduced coverage in exchange markets 2014-2018. Physicians for Fair Coverage. Research by *Avalere*, July 2018.
25. Individual markets nationally face high premium increases in coming years absent federal or state action. *Covered California*, March 12, 2018.
26. Pear, R. F.T.C. wary of mergers by hospitals. *New York Times*, September 17, 2014.
27. Wide variation in hospital charges for blood tests called 'irrational.' Capsules. *Kaiser Health News*, August 15, 2014.

28. Kahn, CN. Intolerable risk, irreparable harm: The legacy of physician-owned hospitals. *Health Affairs (Millwood)* 25 (1): 130-133, 2006.

29. Gorman, A. Weak oversight blamed for poor care at California nursing homes going unchecked. *Kaiser Health News*, May 4, 2018.

30. Bernard, TS. Costly rehab for the dying is on the rise at nursing homes, study says. *New York Times*, October 12, 2018.

31. Mahr, J. Understaffed nursing homes face hefty fines under newly passed Illinois legislation. *Chicago Tribune*, June 4, 2019.

32. Cabin, W, Himmelstein, DU, Siman, ML et al. For-profit Medicare home health agencies' costs appear higher and quality appears lower compared to not-for-profit agencies. *Health Affairs* 33 (8): 1460-1465, 2014.

33. Ivory, D, Protess, B, Daniel, J. When you dial 911 and Wall Street answers. *New York Times,* June 25, 2016.

34. Brown, LD. In Stevens, RA, Rosenberg, CE, Burns, LR. (eds). *History and Health Policy in the United States: Putting the Past Back In.* New Brunswick, NJ, *Rutgers University Press*, 2006, p. 46.

CHAPTER 7

INADEQUATE INSURANCE PROTECTION

Most of us fear getting stuck in the river Styx: not on shore among the living, but not dead yet. And most of us will need "help" during that journey, perhaps long before the journey starts.
—Joan Retsinas, sociologist and health care journalist [1]

As we saw in the last chapter, the mission of our corporatized, privatized market-based system is focused on profits, not public needs. Long-term care falls through the cracks as a societal need that all of us will encounter along the way.

This chapter has two goals: (1) to review the many ways by which American seniors, even when insured, find their coverage inadequate when it comes to their needing to pay for LTC; and (2) to briefly discuss the adverse impacts of this shortfall on vulnerable, often frail seniors.

How Health Insurance Fails to Cover Long-Term Care

As we recall from Chapter 1, more than one-half of U. S. seniors will need nursing home or other LTC services in their later years. (Figure 1.2, page 7). The costs of this care have become unaffordable for those with middle or low incomes, leaving all but the wealthy to depend on some kind of a safety net. That raises the question whether or not the U. S. can set a high enough priority to develop a national plan to ensure a safety net for long-term care, when it has yet to do so.

Private health insurance

Joan Retsinas, of the opening quote, asks an important, still unresolved question: "The last journey: who will pay?" The answer today is—neither the private sector, as long-term care insurance goes away, nor the government, except through Medicaid if the recipient becomes eligible by spending down to poverty. As she points out, LTC ranges from 24-hour monitoring to occasional meals, from nurses and home health aides to unpaid family members, and from elevators to ramps. All of which costs more money than most people have (often more than $100,000 a year), and takes more help than many family members can provide. [2] Figure 7.1 indicates the projected spending on long-term care for the more than one-half of Americans who will end up needing that care. [3]

FIGURE 7.1

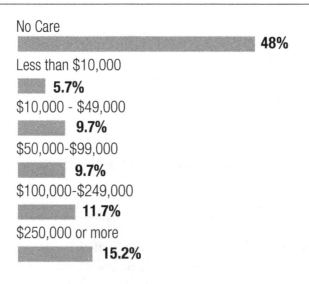

PROJECTED SPENDING ON NEEDED LONG-TERM CARE

No Care
48%

Less than $10,000
5.7%

$10,000 - $49,000
9.7%

$50,000-$99,000
9.7%

$100,000-$249,000
11.7%

$250,000 or more
15.2%

Source: Department of Health and Human Services

The costs of private health insurance are going out of sight, even as its coverage is decreasing. A recent analysis by Modern Healthcare of the U. S. Bureau of Labor Statistics' data found that the Consumer Price Index (CPI) for health insurance spiked 10.7 percent in April 2019 over the previous 12 months. That increase dwarfed the CPI for medical services over that 12-month period, which rose by 2.3 percent, compared to overall inflation going up by 2 percent. That made Wall Street investors happy as profits of the eight largest publicly traded insurers posted net income of $9.3 billion in the first quarter of 2019, an increase of almost 30 percent.[4] Figure 7.2 shows the meteoric climb in the costs of health insurance in recent years.

FIGURE 7.2

METEORIC CLIMB IN THE COST OF HEALTH INSURANCE, 2014 - 2019

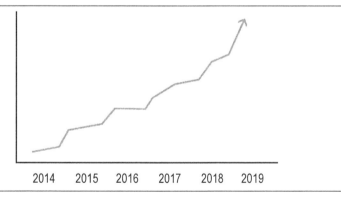

Source: Livingston, S., Health insurance inflation hits highest point in five years. *Modern Healthcare*, May 17, 2019

Long-term care insurance

Long-term care insurance has almost become a relic of history. Private insurers soon found that their initial expectation that big profits would come from healthier young people attracted to low premiums, with many dropping out, went away as LTC costs and claims spiraled upward. Enrollees who expected real protection instead encountered steep premium increases and restricted benefits, such as waiting periods before benefits would occur and exclusions for dementia. The number of insurers offering such policies fell from 125 in 2002 to just 15 in 2014. [5]

Employer sponsored insurance

Employer-based health insurance has a long history in this country, dating back to World War II when employers needed to attract workers without violating wartime wage controls. It spread rapidly after the war, and about 160 million people are so covered today.

But there are chinks in the armor of that coverage. A recent analysis of employer-based insurance by the *Los Angeles Times* has found that soaring deductibles and medical bills have pushed millions of insured middle class Americans to the breaking point. Annual deductibles have gone up by almost four-fold in the last 12 years. Four in ten people with job-based insurance report that they don't have enough savings to cover the deductible, while one in six say they have had to take an extra job, cut back on food, or move in with friends or family. [6] A 2019 report from the Commonwealth Fund estimated that 23.6 million Americans with employer-based insurance had high premium contributions or high out-of-pocket costs for health care relative to income, or both. [7]

People with employer-based health insurance now fare worse than those insured through the ACAs marketplace. Low-income families (below twice the poverty level) with employer-based insurance are spending 14 percent of their income on premiums and out-of-pocket costs compared to their counterparts with ACA coverage, who spend 8.4 percent of their income on these items. Drew Altman, President and CEO of the Kaiser Family Foundation, summed up the problem this way:

> *Employer-based coverage is by far the largest source of health insurance, and it now provides the least financial protection for lower income workers who need it most. We debate affordability of the ACA marketplaces a lot, but we don't talk about this far larger problem much, if at all.* [8]

Compliant vs. non-compliant ACA plans

Although the GOP and Trump administration failed to repeal the ACA on multiple occasions over the last three years, they did effectively sabotage it in a number of ways. The individual mandate was repealed as part of the 2017 GOP tax cut bill. [9] Seema Verma, as CMS head, issued a 365-page rule in October 2017 allowing states to determine how the ACA's essential benefits should be defined, relaxed the threshold for state regulators to review premium increases, and let insurers spend more of their premium revenues on profits and administration. [10]

In later moves, CMS has granted waivers to many states that allow them to offer skimpier, cheaper plans that evade the ACA's requirements, such as patient protections of pre-existing conditions and coverage of ten essential benefits. [11] As a result of these state waivers, short-term limited benefit plans, renewable for up to three years, are being widely marketed. They are bare bones at most, will draw healthier people out of the risk pool, will be highly profitable for insurers but increase premiums for ACA-compliant plans which will end up with older, sicker enrollees. This major change prompted Dean Baker, co-director of the Center for Economic and Policy Research, to this observation:

> *A couple earning $65,000 a year could easily find themselves paying more than half of their after-tax income for insurance premiums. And they could still find themselves liable for thousands of dollars in health care expenses.* [12]

A recent analysis by the Commonwealth Fund of laws and regulations affecting short-term plans in nine states and the District of Columbia revealed some interesting examples of how unprotected enrollees are in these supposed "insurance" plans. Their attractively low premiums may draw many people to them vs. ACA marketplace plans, but they end up as "bait and switch" when it comes to any real protection. Table 7.1 compares an ACA plan with a short-term plan in Dallas, Texas. [13]

TABLE 7.1

COMPARISON OF MARKETPLACE PLANS TO SHORT-TERM PLANS FOR SALE IN DALLAS, TEXAS

Benefit design	ACA-compliant plans	Short-term plans
Highest deductible	$7,900	$25,000
Limit on total covered benefits	None	$100,000–$2,000,000 per contract term
Available regardless of health status	Yes	No, except one insurer offering guaranteed options with a $100,000 limit in total coverage per contract term
Preexisting conditions	Covered	Excluded
Mental health and substance use	Covered in parity with other services	Excluded by three of six insurers analyzed; all three insurers covering mental health and substance use treatment limit outpatient visits to 10 visits at $50 and limit inpatient services to $100 per day for these categories
Outpatient prescription drugs	Covered	Excluded by five of six insurers analyzed; only insurer covering outpatient prescription drugs limits coverage to $3,000 and excludes prescription drugs in lower-cost plans
Pregnancy and delivery	Covered	Excluded

Source: Palanker D, Kona M, Curran E. States step up to protect insurance markets and consumers from short-term health plans. *The Commonwealth Fund*, May 2, 2019

Public health insurance
Medicare

Traditional Medicare provides no coverage for the needs of seniors needing LTC beyond initial short-term coverage of patients in nursing homes for initial stabilization and rehabilitation treatments after being hospitalized. When seniors attempt to gain further coverage beyond Medicare through Part F Medigap policies, they find that insurers can deny this coverage based on pre-existing conditions in all but four states. [14]

Medicaid

Medicaid is the current final lifeline for covering LTC. Enacted in 1965 under the Lyndon Johnson administration as a social insurance program to provide lower-income Americans with the health care they need, it has become a mainstay for assuring necessary medical care for about 74 million Americans. It covers one in five Americans, almost one-half of all births, 39 percent of children, more than one-quarter of mental health services, and about two-thirds of nursing home and LTC services. [15]

Although Medicaid provides the main coverage for LTC, its coverage varies widely from state to state and our safety net remains fragile. It is a target for deficit-minded conservatives in federal and state legislatures for reduction of the deficit on the backs of vulnerable Americans. Red states continue to search for ways to limit their Medicaid programs, sometimes aided by federal waivers. [16] Some states are very restrictive in their eligibility for Medicaid coverage of long-term care.

In the 14 states that did not expand Medicaid under the ACA, 2.5 million adults have fallen into a coverage gap by earning too much to qualify for Medicaid but not enough to qualify for subsidies under the ACA. [17] Two Medicaid-related initiatives, which have provided matching funds to states to help seniors and disabled persons transition from institutional to community-based care since 2007, are scheduled to expire unless reauthorized by Congress by the end of 2019. [18]

Impacts of inadequate coverage

These are some of the adverse impacts on those needing LTC when their health insurance falls way short of their needs.

1. Loss of long-term care insurance

Long-term care often costs more than $100,000 a year. Although in the past one could prepare for these costs by purchasing long-term care insurance, this industry is dying due to high and increasing costs of care for those who end up in nursing homes, assisted living, or at home. This couple found how insecure this kind of insurance has become:

> *David and Sally Wylie, retired in their late 60s on Vinalhaven Island in Maine, had long-term care insurance for the last ten years. Over that period, the cost of their insurance through CNA Financial Corp. increased by more than 90 percent, putting a severe strain on their budget.* [19]

2. Medicare Advantage plan refused to pay

Here is one couple's bad experience with privatized Medicare Advantage:

> *John McAuliff, 77, and his wife, Ann, 78, in Charlotte, North Carolina, were satisfied with their Medicare Advantage plan until she had a severe stroke in 2017. Their insurer refused to pay for further care after several months. While the couple challenged the denial and finally prevailed in a hearing before an administrative law judge, they went back to traditional Medicare and fortunately also obtained a supplemental Medigap policy which together covered all their medical expenses.* [20]

They were lucky to get Medigap after this kind of experience, since seniors are often denied such a policy because of pre-existing conditions. [21]

3. Insurance stops paying in a nursing home

This patient's story illustrates how precarious his protection was when he became too sick for a private payer to continue coverage.

> *Alan Shoen, after two hospitalizations after a fall and later with a bladder infection and pancreatitis, was told that his insurance would soon stop paying and that he should move to an assisted living facility, where he would receive less care. As he said at the time, "They are running a business. I get that, but it seems they forget the patient element in all of this."* [22]

4. Exhausting personal and family resources

Because we lack an adequate national policy to pay for the increasing needs of our aging population needing long-term care, we force most patients and their families to exhaust their financial resources as they cope with paying for LTC. Here is one such example:

Ms. S prepared well for her later years. She saved carefully, bought a long-term care policy, and retired with more than $600,000. By the time she died at 94, however, she had been in a nursing home for five years, was on Medicaid, and had gone through all of her savings. [23]

5. Filing for bankruptcy

With 30 million uninsured and more than 80 million under-insured, Americans were forced to borrow $88 billion in 2019 to pay for their health care costs. As those costs continue to soar with no end in sight, 530,000 families are forced into bankruptcy each year, two-thirds of which are due to illness and medical bills when they can no longer afford essential health care. Dr. David Himmel-stein, internist, health policy expert, and co-founder of Physicians for a National Health Program (PNHP), describes the problem this way:

> *Unless you're Bill Gates, you're just one serious illness away from bankruptcy. For middle-class Americans, health insurance offers little protection. Most of us have policies with so many loopholes, copayments, and deductibles that illness can put you in the poorhouse. And even the best job-based insurance often vanishes when prolonged illness causes job loss—just when families need it most.*[24]

Private health insurance through our current multi-payer system of some 1,300 insurers makes it next to impossible to provide coverage to people in their later years when they come to require LTC. In their goal to maximize revenue, private insurers select lower-risk enrollees and often dis-enroll sicker people needing too much expensive care. Under the "20-80 rule," 20 percent of the population accounts for 80 percent of all health care spending, while just 5 percent uses almost one-half of total spending. [25] The unavoidable mathematics of risk pools therefore needs a different kind of insurance—universal coverage through not-for-profit social insurance in the public sector, which spreads risk across the largest possible risk pool, ideally our entire population of some 326 million Americans.

Unfortunately, neither the private sector nor government are stepping up to cover LTC, but are also making it even more difficult for seniors to gain such coverage. CMS is promoting further privatization of both Medicare and Medicaid as efforts to impede the ACA continue. State waivers have been especially controversial, with many states fighting back, with broad bipartisan support, against the loss of the ACA's patient protections. [26] Congressional Democrats have also joined this effort by attempting to block the adverse impacts of these state waivers that avoid ACA patient protections. Meanwhile, the pending lawsuit filed by Texas and 17 other GOP-led states, joined also by the Department of Justice, claiming that the ACA is unconstitutional, is still unresolved.

Conclusion

We are now seeing a battle over the nation's safety net for health care and the extent to which the government, at both federal and state levels, should intervene to assure access to affordable care. With a GOP controlled Senate and a Trump presidency, state block grants threaten that both levels of government will cut back the safety net, already shredded, even further. All this comes at a time when the U. S. is seeing growing inequities and worse health outcomes despite spending far more on health care than other advanced countries around the world.

We are therefor left with a stark reality—few among us are wealthy enough to pay for LTC in our future time of need, so must look to spending down to poverty to get Medicaid coverage until we can enact universal coverage through Medicare for All (H. R. 1384 in the House bill).

We will revisit how to address the lack of insurance protection for LTC in Part III, when we will start with financing reform to gain equitable, affordable coverage for this essential care. But for now, we need to move on to the next chapter, where we will consider why LTC continues to be devalued within our society.

References:

1.	Retsinas, J. The last journey: Who will pay? *The Progressive Populist*, June 15, 2019, p. 15.
2.	Ibid # 1.
3.	Scism, L. Safety net frays for millions of retirees. *Wall Street Journal*, January 18, 2018: A1.
4.	Livingston, S. Health insurance inflation hits highest point in five years. *Modern Healthcare,* May 17, 2019.
5.	Ibid # 1.
6.	Levey, NN. Health insurance deductibles soar, leaving Americans with unaffordable bills. *Los Angeles Times*, May 2, 2019.
7.	Hayes, SL, Collins, SR, Radley, DC. How much U. S. households with employer insurance spend on premiums and out-of-pocket costs: A state-by-state look. *The Commonwealth Fund*, May 23, 2019.
8.	Altman, D. For low-income people, employer health coverage is worse than ACA. *Axios*, April 15, 2019.
9.	Meyer, H, Livingston, S, Dickson, V. CMS to allow states to define essential benefits. *Modern Healthcare*, October 29, 2017.
10.	Verma, S, as quoted by, Lighty, M. New Medicaid work requirements will deny more care. *Sanders Institute*, November 15, 2017.
11.	Hackman, M. States can waive more ACA rules. *Wall Street Journal*, October 23, 2018.
12.	Baker, D. Trump succeeds in making insurance for people with health problems unaffordable. *The Progressive Populist*, October 1, 2018, p. 11.
13.	Palanker, D, Kona, M, Curran, E. States step up to protect insurance markets and consumers from short-term health plans. *The Commonwealth Fund*, May 2, 2019.
14.	Boccuti, C, Jacobson, G, Orgera, K et al. Medigap enrollment and consumer protections vary across states. Issue Brief. *Kaiser Family Foundation*, July 11, 2018.
15.	Galewitz, P. Medicaid covers all that? It's the backstop of America's ailing health care system. *Kaiser Health News*, September 25, 2017.
16.	Baker, S. Red states' Medicaid gamble: Paying more to cover fewer people. *Axios*, April 17, 2019. 17.
17.	Garfield, R, Orgera, K, Damico, A. The coverage gap: Uninsured poor adults in states that do not expand Medicaid. *Kaiser Family Foundation*, March 2019.

18. Lee, C. Two Medicaid-related initiatives that help promote long-term care at home and in the community, rather than institutions, are set to expire at the end of December. *Kaiser Family Foundation*, November 25, 2019.

19. Ibid #3.

20. Pear, R. Trump administration peppers inboxes with plugs for private Medicare plans. *New York Times*, December 1, 2018.

21. KFF Newsroom. In all but four states, seniors on Medicare can be denied a Medigap policy due to pre-existing conditions, except during windows of opportunity. July 11, 2018.

22. Bernard, TS, Pear, R. Complaints about nursing home evictions rise, and regulators take note. *New York Times,* February 22, 2018.

23. Lieber, R. One woman's slide from middle class to Medicaid. Your Money Column. *New York Times*, July 7, 2017.

24. Himmelstein, DU, Lawless, RM, Thorne, D et al. Medical bankruptcy: Still common despite the Affordable Care Act. *Am J Public Health*, March 2019.

25. National Institute for Health Care Management. A comparatively small number of sick people account for most health care spending. August 2, 2012.

26. DeBonis, M. House passes measure to block ACA waivers to states. *The Washington Post*, May 10, 2019.

CHAPTER 8

UNDER VALUATION OF LONG-TERM CARE

As we saw in Chapter 1, caregivers for LTC are themselves a vulnerable group—mostly women earning close to or below the minimum wage, uninsured without sick leave, and often dependent on food stamps and Medicaid to support their own families. As we have also seen, we have a huge shortage of caregivers in this country. Their work is hard, requires personal relationship skills, and often high-risk, especially when it becomes necessary to lift and move patients much bigger and heavier than themselves.

This chapter has two goals: (1) to consider how LTC has been devalued over so many years leading to the growing crisis in providing these essential services; and (2) to briefly discuss how this crisis has occurred with so little appreciation for its gravity among the public and policy makers.

How Long-Term Care Is Undervalued

Here are some of the many ways that LTC is devalued in the U. S.

1. Underpaid and undervalued

This is what Roxanne Trigg, a home health aide in Milwaukee, Wisconsin, has to cope with as one typical example of how underpaid LTC caregivers are in this country.

I work hard at a demanding job, seven days a week. I save taxpayers money and bring comfort and dignity to a person with a severe disability, yet my family is living in poverty.

I work for a for-profit home care company. After five years, I make just $9.15 an hour, with no sick leave and no *vacation. It used to be $9.00 an hour but then the agency told us a raise was coming. It turned out to be just 15 cents, which was just humiliating. Living on $9.15 an hour means choosing which bill to pay and which one to be late on, even if it means you have to pay a penalty later. A few months ago, I had to risk getting our lights turned off by not paying the bill so I could buy shoes and clothes for the two grandkids I take care of. My paycheck doesn't get bigger every year, but my grandkids do.*

I love my job. But I am the sole supporter of my family and I'm paid so little that we can't cover our expenses. It's just wrong. [1]

Sylvia Foon Sau Liange, in Seattle, Washington, has a similar story. Her husband died of leukemia, leaving her a single mother providing care for her adult son with autism, as well as for an 86-year-woman with dementia. As she says about her work:

People in the outside world barely notice the work we do. The families see it. Our clients see it and they appreciate it. But every day is a struggle to figure out how to make my paycheck stretch to fit all the things I need to support my son. It just doesn't seem right that we do so much but get paid so little. [2]

2. Near Poverty wages

Median annual incomes for nearly 2 million home care workers, working full time, are just $16,200, close to the federal poverty level. While their wages are not declining, they remain inadequate to meet their basic needs, since they have unpredictable and part-time hours that reduce their earnings. Since the number of hours of needed care often vary widely, caregivers typically work for multiple clients and face an ongoing challenge of patching together full-time, steady work. Because of this, only two in five home caregivers are able to work full-time, year round. With their low incomes, home caregivers all face the burden of paying for their rental housing, food, utilities, child care expenses, and health care.[3]

Home caregivers often give up successful careers in other areas to take on care of their aging family members, thereby increasing the burden of providing for their own families. That is what happened for Alantris Muhammad in Chicago, Illinois:

> *I've been working in home care now. I provide full-time care for my mother. I left my career in insurance so that my mom could continue to live at home with family. It was a hard decision to make, but without a home care worker my mother would be forced into a nursing home because she needs a caregiver around the clock.*
>
> *I've raised five sons and I'm currently putting the fourth through college. Workers like me face tough decisions all the time—should we pay the tuition bill or fix the oven that broke right before Thanksgiving? Can we put gas in the car to take our clients to medical appointments or do we need to save that money for groceries?* [4]

3. More than one-half of home health aides rely on some form of public benefits

In order to make ends meet, more than one-half of home care workers rely on such public assistance programs as Medicaid, food stamps, and housing and heating assistance. Four in ten home care aides earn less than 133 percent of the federal poverty level, making them eligible for expanded Medicaid under the ACA. [5]

4. Misunderstanding that LTC is unskilled work.

Here is Theresa King's story that makes the case that LTC caregiving is by no means unskilled.

> *I care for an energetic 87-year old woman with Alzheimer's disease. I'm responsible for everything from making sure she takes her medication to preparing her food, and helping her with dressing, bathing, and toileting.*
>
> *These are the everyday tasks that most of us take for granted, but seniors and people with disabilities couldn't manage without home care workers.*

It takes love, patience, and understanding to do this job well. It requires organizational skills and a lot of physical strength and hard work.

I make $10 an hour, just a dollar over the state minimum wage. No matter how hard I try I can never get anywhere near full-time hours, and that still wouldn't be enough. It shouldn't be this way.

None of us are looking to get rich—we just want to be able to live and support our families like everyone else. [6]

5. Exclusion from Fair Labor Standards Act (FLSA)

The FLSA has excluded home care aides from federal minimum wage and overtime laws since its inception in 1938. Fortunately, however, the U. S. Department of Labor issued a new rule, effective January 1, 2015, that extended minimum wage and overtime protections to almost 2 million home health care care workers who care for the elderly, ill, and disabled. [7]

6. Lack of paid sick leave

Sick leave is almost never available for home caregivers. When they get the flu, they face a double whammy—making their already precarious financial situation worse while not wanting to risk going to work sick and infecting their client. The physical labor of their work is hard, and sometimes even backbreaking. In 2010, for example, the rate of on-the-job injuries for home health aides resulting in missed work was about twice that of the labor force overall. [8] Yet, these workers have no protections from illness or injury.

7. Uninsured or underinsured

Wendy Matney, 39-year-old home health aide, hesitated to tell her family not to call 911. She has a form of epilepsy that causes frequent, sometimes violent, seizures. She had enough trips to the hospital to know that each trip results in thousands of dollars in medical bills under the *family's high deductible health plan. She and her husband are struggling with more than $20,000 in medical debt, and cannot afford more. Hit with a lawsuit over unpaid bills, they are declaring bankruptcy, giving up hope of moving out of their trailer and buying a house.* [9]

8. Lack of career advancement opportunities

There are two formal occupations being tracked by the U.S. Department of Labor—home health aides and personal care aides. According to federal definitions, *home health aides* provide "routine individualized health care such as changing bandages and dressing wounds, and applying topical medications to the elderly, convalescents, or persons with disabilities at the patient's home or in a care facility. Monitor or report changes in health status. May also provide personal care such as bathing, dressing, and grooming the patients."

Personal care aides "assist the elderly, convalescents, or persons with disabilities with daily living activities in the person's home or in a care facility. Duties performed at a place of residence may include keeping house (making beds, doing the laundry, washing dishes) and preparing meals. May provide assistance at non-residential care facilities. May advise families, the elderly, convalescents, and persons with disabilities regarding such things as nutrition, cleanliness, and household activities." [10]

Both occupations are expected to grow by almost 50 percent between 2012 and 2022, but formal training is still minimal and there is no organized pathway for career advancement.

Why Has the Crisis in Long-Term Care Happened?

1. Apathy among the public and policy makers

Long-term care services have long been under recognized and under appreciated, except among those receiving such care. As Henry Moss, author of the excellent book *The 2030 Caregiving Crisis: A Heavy Burden for Boomer Children,* says:

*Long-term care is the personal care we need when
chronic illness, physical disability, cognitive impairment,
mental illness, or frailty makes us unable to safely carry
out our normal activities of daily living, including toileting,
grooming, dressing, bathing, feeding, and moving about. It
may also include shopping, personal finance, cooking, trav-
el, and general housekeeping, along with assistive technolo-
gy, home modifications, and certain social services. . . . It is,
therefore, certainly part of health care.* [11]

2. Demographic changes

As we saw in Chapter 1, the U. S. population is aging faster
than most of us realize, with seniors projected to outnumber children under the age of 18 by 2035, for the first time in the nation's
history. Baby boomers, born between 1946 and 1964, are living
longer and reshaping America's elderly population.

We can, and should, now change our previous understanding
of the human life cycle. Dr. Louise Aronson, geriatrician, professor of medicine at the University of California San Francisco, and
author of the just-published book, *Elderhood: Redefining Aging,
Transforming Medicine, Reimagining Life*, suggests a new way to
look at elderhood as the last chapter in a revised life cycle with its
expected phases of independence and dependence. (Figure 8.1) [12]

3. Low wages

The Paraprofessional Healthcare Institute (PHI) gives us this
long historical view as to why LTC caregivers are paid so little:

*The low wages of home care workers are rooted in the
history of exploitation of labor based on race and gender,
particularly the devaluation of women's labor in the household. Because women often do this work for their families
for "free," it isn't considered deserving of the same re-
spect—and wages—offered to workers who are employed
outside the home.*

Thus, the women—and in particular, women of color—who do this work have long suffered from substandard wages. Of home care workers, 89 percent are women, and more than half are people of color. One in four home health aides is an immigrant to the U. S.

Today, home care work and workers remain largely invisible—highly valued by individuals and families who need them but undervalued by society as a whole. As a result, the home care aides who make it possible for millions of elders and people with disabilities to have quality lives at home are not treated like professionals. [13]

FIGURE 8.1

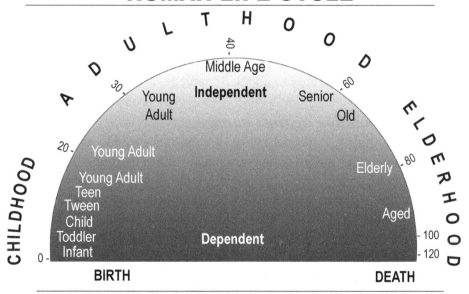

REVISED VERSION OF THE HUMAN LIFE CYCLE

Source: Aronson, L. *Elderhood: Redefining Aging, Transforming Medicine, Reimagining Life*, New York, *Bloomsbury Publishing*, 2019, p. 270

4. Lack of job benefits

Without any employer-based health insurance or paid sick leave, home caregivers are especially vulnerable themselves. They have to deal with their own health problems, including chronic conditions and injuries, and usually cannot afford preventive care. Fortunately, however, almost one-half of them qualify for Medicaid.

5. High turnover of caregivers

Because of their low wages and lack of job-based benefits, one-half of the LTC workforce turns over each year, thereby disrupting the continuity of relationships essential to LTC. Some caregivers have to leave because they can't afford to stay. That creates a revolving door of caregivers, with ongoing difficult challenges to recruit their replacements.

In order to address the recruitment problem, some states have funded programs that provide coverage for personal care and home health aides' care to family member caregivers. California's In-Home Supportive Services Program, the largest in the country, extends this coverage to three in four family caregivers, and has reduced the turnover rate to about 30 percent. [14]

6. Discrimination against immigrants

According to a recent study, immigrants provide a disproportionate amount of LTC, accounting for more than one-quarter of formal and non-formal direct caregiving. Figure 8.2 shows the percentage of direct care workers in nursing homes in 2017 by nativity status. [15]

Although the U. S. has an increasing need for LTC workers, many of whom are immigrants, current immigration policies pose a barrier to this need being filled. The Trump administration has drastically reduced the numbers of immigrants entering the country, with a focus on "skilled immigrants," thereby raising the bar for LTC caregiver recruitment. [16] Here again, however, California has taken the lead in granting access for undocumented immigrants to drivers' licenses, in-state tuition, university grants, student loans, professional licenses, and just recently, to enrollment in Medi-Cal, the state's Medicaid program, for unauthorized immigrants under age 26. [17]

FIGURE 8.2

PERCENT OF DIRECT CARE WORKERS AND HOUSEKEEPING, CONSTRUCTION, AND MAINTAINANCE STAFF IN NURSING HOMES, BY NATIVITY STATUS, 2017

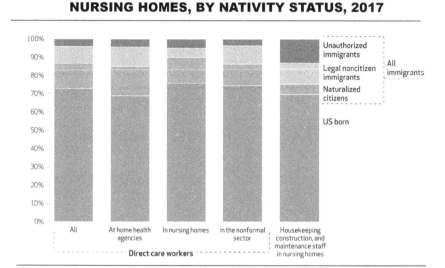

Source: Zallman, L. Finnegan, KE, Himmelstein, DU et al. *Health Affairs* 38(6): 924, 2019

7. Lack of political power to unionize

For many years, LTC caregivers have not had enough political capital or economic power to demand higher wages and improved employment conditions. That, fortunately, is starting to change. Here is the story of one caregiver in St. Paul, Minnesota, Sumer Spika, becoming an activist for much needed change.

> *Sumer cares for a little girl, Jayla, who has Opitz Syndrome and is at constant risk of choking due to breathing and swallowing problems. She is also deaf, so that they use sign language to communicate. Sumer has seen both wage and benefit cuts over the last four years. In response, she and her co-workers in Minnesota's home care program voted to form a union.* [18]

Conclusion

We will return to this subject in Chapter 11 of Part III and address how the problems discussed here can be dealt with in the future. For now, it is time to turn to the next chapter, which has much to do with what has brought us to this sad state of affairs in long-term care.

References:

1. *How poverty wages undermine home care in America*, New York, NY. 2015, *Paying the Price,* Paraprofessional Healthcare Institute, Bronx, New York, February, 2015, p. 4.
2. Ibid # 1, p. 15.
3. Campbell, S. *Direct care worker wages are increasing but challenges persist.* Paraprofessional Healthcare Institute (PHI) National, September 30, 2019. Ibid # 1, p. 15.
4. Ibid # 1, p. 7.
5. Ibid # 1, p. 8.
6. Ibid # 1, p. 2.
7. Home health care workers now protected under the Fair Labor Standards Act (FLSA). U. S. Department of Labor, September 18, 2013.
8. Ibid # 1, p. 12.
9. Levey, NN. Soaring insurance deductibles and high drug prices hit sick Americans with a 'double whammy,' *Los Angeles Times,* June 6, 2019.
10. U. S. Bureau of Labor Statistics, February 2010.
11. Moss, H. Long-term care and Medicare for All: An interview with PNHP NY Metro's Henry Moss, 2019.
12. Aronson, L. *Elderhood: Redefining Aging, Transforming Medicine, Reimagining Life.* New York. *Bloomsbury Publishing,* 2019, p. 270.
13. Ibid # 1, p. 11.
14. Ibid # 1, p. 3.
15. Zallman, L, Finnegan, KE, Himmelstein, DU et al. Care for America's elderly and disabled people relies on immigrant labor. *Health Affairs* 38 (6): 919-926, 2019.
16. Ibid # 14.
17. Lazo, A. California budget expands health care for immigrants. *Wall Street Journal,* June 15-16, 2019: A 4.
18. Ibid # 1, p. 14.

CHAPTER 9

CONSERVATIVE TAX POLICIES vs. THE COMMON GOOD

Government is instituted for the common good; for the protection, safety, prosperity and happiness of the people; and not for the profit, honor, or private interest of any one man, family or class of men.

—John Adams, one of our founding fathers
and second president of the United States [1]

The issue of universal coverage is not a matter of economics. Little more than 1 percent of GDP assigned to health could cover it all. It is a matter of soul.

—Uwe E. Reinhardt, Ph.D., the late Professor of Political Economy
and Public Affairs at Princeton University and author of *Priced Out:
The Economic and Ethical Costs of American Health Care.* [2]

We have seen in earlier chapters how U. S. health care policy is dominated by powerful market forces as our "system" has become increasingly corporatized and consolidated. Health care has become just another commodity for sale in an unfettered marketplace as privatization of public programs, promoted by GOP legislators and policy makers, has steadily grown. Disparities and inequities have increased, and the battle lines have been more sharply drawn between advocates of reform for the common good vs. corporate stakeholders and their investors on Wall Street.

Meanwhile there has been a steady push by conservatives to challenge the social contract of Medicare and Medicaid, enacted in the mid-1960s. In so doing, they have disparaged these programs as entitlements and welfare programs not within the ongoing responsibility of government.

This chapter has two goals: (1) to bring historical context to the unresolved battle over tax policy and the role of government in U. S. health care; and (2) to briefly discuss the values that determine future directions, especially the extent to which government should be involved in ensuring access to affordable health care, including long-term care.

Historical Overview of Tax Policy

There has been a long-standing tug of war for more than 100 years in this country between Democrats favoring tax fairness and Republicans favoring the wealthy. Theodore Roosevelt complained in 1910 about "swollen fortunes for the few." Under the New Deal of President Franklin D. Roosevelt, tax rates were increased in 1935 by up to 75 percent for the wealthiest Americans. President Reagan went to the other extreme in 1980, dropping the top income tax rate to 28%. Since then, incomes among the top 1% have soared compared to the rest of the population. The richest 0.1% now own 19 percent of national wealth, about three times the concentration in the late 1970s and approaching the levels of the late 1920s. [3]

Figure 9.1 shows the average tax rate for the top 0.1 % and the bottom 90 % of income earners since 1913. Interestingly, the bottom group has paid almost as high a tax rate as the top group over the last 40 years. [4]

The GOP has long waged war against "entitlement programs" through its tax policies, which continue to favor the wealthy over the needs of the most vulnerable among us, while also raising the questions of deservedness. Both Medicare and Medicaid were passed in the mid-1960s as social insurance programs, for those age 65 and over and for lower-income Americans, respectively. Supporters of more recent regressive tax policies tend to perpetuate an unfounded belief that those needing Medicaid are lazy or otherwise undeserving of help, ignoring the fact that they are mostly already working and unable to afford essential health care. [5]

That battle has accelerated under the Trump administration. After multiple failed attempts by the GOP to repeal the ACA, they finally passed the December 2017 tax bill, which repealed the individual mandate, led to an increase in the number of uninsured, and raised the federal deficit to an estimated $1.45 trillion. Since Medicare and Medicaid account for about 30 percent of the federal budget, they have been increasingly targeted for future cutbacks under the guise of reducing the federal deficit, which has increased during the Trump years. [6]

FIGURE 9.1

AVERAGE TAX RATES FOR THE TOP 0.1% VS. BOTTOM 90%, 1913-2020

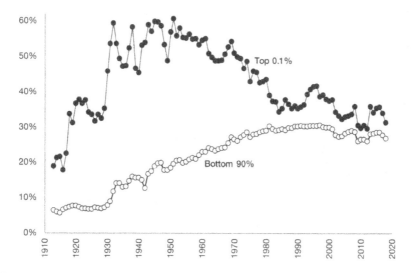

Source: Saez, E, Zucman, G. *The Triumph of Injustice: How the Rich Dodge Taxes and How to Make Them Pay.* New York. *W. W. Norton & Company,* 2019, p. 42.

Trump's latest intent to shrink Medicaid is to redefine how poverty is defined through a proposed "chained consumer price index," which if adopted, will most likely transfer millions of people previously eligible for Medicaid to the rolls of the ineligible though still living in poverty. [7]

In February 2018, Congress passed the 2018 Bipartisan Budget Act, which increased military spending at the expense of large cuts in Medicare funding for long-term care. [8] That same month, Trump proposed a budget for 2019 that would eliminate Medicaid expansion under the ACA, transfer the rest of Medicaid into a system of capped payments to states, and expand work requirements for Medicaid eligibility. [9]

In October 2018, the Republican-controlled Congress quietly passed Trump's budget for FY 2019, which gave a big tax handout to the wealthiest Americans, and cut the U. S. corporate tax rate from 35 to 21 percent, leading not to trickle down job creation but to corporate stock buybacks and explosion of the federal deficit. [10] According to the Institute on Taxation and Economic Policy (ITEP), however, large companies in practice over the next year often paid less than that through deductions, tax breaks and other loopholes. In fact, 91 corporations in the Fortune 500 paid no federal taxes in 2018 (including online retailer Amazon), and the average corporate tax rate fell to just 11.3 percent that year, the lowest effective tax rate since ITEP started to record these data back in 1984. [11]

In mid-March 2019, Trump proposed a budget for FY 2020 that would slash federal spending on Medicaid and Medicare by $1.4 trillion and more than $800 billion, respectively, over the coming decade. Many legislators in Congress warned that cuts of this magnitude will create a firestorm of protest from the states when they realize how state block grants or severely capped federal payments for Medicaid will impact them. [12]

Such cuts would threaten America's social contract with lower-income and middle-income Americans that has held since the mid-1960s. Fortunately, these draconian cuts are not likely to become enacted with a Democrat-controlled House, but they reflect Trump's cruel and uncaring values. Wendell Potter, author of the excellent 2010 book, *Deadly Spin: An Insurance Company Insider Speaks Out on How Corporate PR Is Killing and Deceiving Americans*, made this observation about Trump's proposed cuts:

> *It is obvious what he's attempting: Help the special interests loot our tax dollars, and then demand the most vulnerable Americans cover the difference.* [13]

Robert Kuttner, economist and author of *Everything for Sale: The Virtues and Limits of Markets*, summarizes what has happened since the Reagan era in this way:

The era since 1981 has been one of turning away from public remediation, toward tax cuts, limited social spending, deregulation, and privatization. None of this has worked well, except for the very top. For everyone else, the shift to conservative policies generated more economic insecurity.[14]

As we saw in Chapter 6, privatization of public programs, especially of Medicare and Medicaid, has led to increasing corporate profits, further skewing of risk pools, and erosion of Medicaid as the last remaining publicly financed safety net for many millions of vulnerable Americans. This patient's story has become typical of this situation.

Alice Jacobs, 90, once owned a factory and horses. She raised four children and buried two husbands. But years in an assisted living facility drained her savings, and now she relies on Medicaid to pay for her care at Dogwood Village, a nonprofit, county-owned nursing home in Orange, Virginia, where her fellow residents include teachers, farmers, doctors, lawyers, and health aides. As she says, "You think you have enough money to last all your life, and here I am." [15]

The Ongoing Battle over Taxes, Values and the Role of Government

In the aftermath of tax policies of the GOP and Trump administration, inequality of wealth and income has become extreme. Just a few billionaires can now rig the U. S. economy. Wealth of the Walton, Koch, and Mars families have grown by 6,000 percent while the median household wealth of Americans has fallen since 1982. [16] The wealthiest 1% of American households own 40 % of the country's wealth while the bottom 90 % own just 20 %. [17] Given these facts, is there any doubt that tax policies in recent years have been major contributors to the increasing wealth and income gap that divides our nation? While Trump brags on his good economy and argues, without evidence, that his 2017 tax cut trickles down to workers, he fails to acknowledge that this economy continues to generate jobs that won't support a family. [18] Figure 9.2 reminds us to question whether "trickle down" economics actually works, and for whom.

FIGURE 9.2

SANTA CLAUS AND
TRICKLE-DOWN ECONOMICS

"You still believe in trickle-down economics? At you're age?"

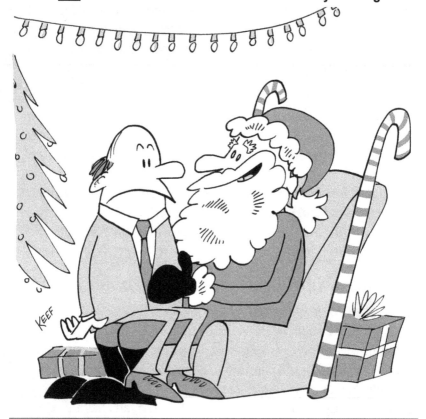

Source: Eric W. Stern, *The New Yorker*, December 23, 2019, p.58

The debate over taxes in past years has focused mainly on the income tax, but we are now starting to hear tax proposals on wealth as well. Democratic presidential candidate Senator Elizabeth Warren has proposed a 2 percent tax on individual and family wealth over $50 million and a 3 percent tax on wealth exceeding

$1 billion. Economist and former U. S. labor secretary Robert Reich notes an important difference between taxing income vs. wealth:

> *Wealth isn't like income. Income is payment for work. Wealth keeps growing automatically and exponentially because it's parked in investments that generate even more wealth. And further: Not only would a wealth tax raise revenue and help bring the economy back into balance, but it would also protect our democracy by reducing the influence of the super-rich on our political system.* [18]

Interestingly, a recent CNBC Millionaire survey has found that 60 percent of millionaires support taxing the wealth of those with more than $50 million in assets. Other polls have shown that 88 percent of Democrats, 62 percent of independents, and 36 percent of Republicans also support a wealth tax. [19]

America's powerful corporations have thrived on GOP tax cuts on the backs of Americans who find increasing barriers to accessing affordable health care. The private health insurance industry and their shareholders are whistling on their way to the bank as they require higher cost sharing from enrollees, impose more restrictive networks, and provide less and less coverage. The numbers of uninsured and underinsured continue to grow as more millions of Americans forgo essential care because of costs and incur worse outcomes. At least 45,000 Americans die each year because of lack of health insurance. [20] Jeffrey Sachs, professor and director of the Center for Sustainable Development at Columbia University, observes:

> *Make no mistake—America's health crisis is the result of greedy corporations and their reckless practices. . . Corporate power has run amok in American politics. Yet the mortality crisis is even worse. The health of the American people depends on restoring democratic oversight and regulation over powerful food and drug companies blinded by greed and arrogance.* [21]

Within the ongoing debate over tax policy during this election season, Emmanuel Saez and Gabriel Zucman, professors of economics at the University of California, Berkeley, ask these important, still unanswered questions in their important new book, *The Triumph of Injustice: How the Rich Dodge Taxes and How to Make Them Pay*:

> *Should billionaires pay 23 % of their income in taxes, as they do in today's America, or closer to 50%, as they did around 1970? Should corporate profits be taxed at 52% as in 1960 or at 21% as they have been since the 2017 tax reform?* [22]

The adverse impacts of GOP and Trump tax policies on the health of Americans cannot be underestimated. They would decimate much of what remains of our safety net for lower and middle-income Americans, especially recipients of Medicaid. As the workhorse of our safety net, Medicaid covers more than 60 percent of nursing home and long-term care expenses, almost one-half of births, more than one-quarter of mental health services, and over one-fifth of substance abuse treatment. [23] As such, it can serve like a canary in the coal mine as an indicator warning of the need for major reform.

That time has already come, but you wouldn't know it from looking at the Trump administration's policies on Medicaid. It is committed to reduce and weaken the ACA's expansion, and cut back eligibility and enrollment through state waivers. More flexibility is being given to the states to manage their own programs with, of course, less federal money. Waivers allow states to impose premiums and cost sharing, work requirements, and/or annual, even lifetime limits. [24] Nine states have already received waivers to impose work requirements for Medicaid recipients despite the failure of this policy in Arkansas, where most targeted people were already working and they just became uninsured. [25]

In 1869, Mark Twain wrote this half-humorous, half-serious open letter to Cornelius Vanderbilt in 1869. Vanderbilt was a self-made millionaire well known for his cutthroat approach to business. He made his first fortune in the steamship business (when he was given the nickname Commodore), then profited from opportunities from the War of 1812, the California Gold rush of 1849, and the Crimean War (1853-1856). Here is Mark Twain's letter, which casts doubt on how much progress has been made in business "ethics" since the 1800s:

> *You observe that I don't say anything about your soul, Vanderbilt. It is because I have evidence that you haven't any. It would be impossible to convince me that a man of your matchless financial ability would overlook so dazzling an "operation," if you had a soul to save, as the purchasing of millions of years of Paradise, and rest, and peace, and pleasure, for so trifling a sum as ten years blamelessly lived on earth—for you probably don't have longer than that to live now, you know, you are very old. Well, I don't know, after all, Vanderbilt—I know you well. You will try to get the price cheaper. You will want those millions of years of rest and pleasure, and you will try to make the trade and get the superb stock; but you will wait till you are on your death-bed, and then offer an hour and forty minutes for it.* [26]

Fast forward to our times, the values represented by the America of the mid-1930s (Social Security) and 1960s (Medicare and Medicaid) give us a model of egalitarian values of caring for all of us through responsive government concerned with societal needs. These values, drawn from the more recent years of this country, give us a useful (or better yet mandatory!) guide to how we should address the increasingly serious problems of our health care system as the political debates over health care fire up again during the 2020 election cycle.

With health care the # 1 issue, the big question today is to decide whether our national health policy should be about private money or public caring. Should the purpose of government be to protect the wealth of the 1% or to serve the common good? The answer in recent decades has been the former, but that will no longer do.

In their recent report, *Poor People's Moral Budget: Everybody Has a Right to Live*, Rev. Drs. William Barber and Liz Theoharis bring us back to how current national priorities and tax policies take our safety net apart:

> *As Rev. Dr. Martin Luther King Jr. has suggested, our state and national budgets prove that many of our elected leaders and their lobbyists treasure the military, corporate tax cuts, and welfare for the wealthy while they give rugged individualism, shame and blame, unfair wages, and a shredded social safety net to the poor. . . . This is a willful act of policy violence at a time when there are 140 million poor and low-income people—over 43.5 percent of the population—in the richest country in the history of the world.* [27]

Conclusion

At this writing, Republicans still have no health care plan of their own and Democratic presidential candidates are split over whether or not to support universal coverage through Medicare for All. The current political debate will determine whether America still has the soul of earlier years.

Many, if not most health economists in this country, still tout the magic of competition in the marketplace to effectively deal with access, cost, and quality issues in health care. That has been tried for decades, and simply does not work, as shown by our increasing crisis in health care despite incremental reform attempts. It is time for bipartisan legislative action at the national level to change how we finance care for the common good. In the next chapter, we will describe how this can be done through financing reform.

References

1.   Adams, J, as quoted by Hartmann, TA. A red privatization story. *The Progressive Populist*, November 15, 2014, p. 11.
2.   Reinhardt, U. As quoted by McCanne, D. Quote of the Day, November 15, 2017.
3.   Rubin, R. The next tax revolution? *Wall Street Journal*, February 16-17, 2019: C 1, C2.
4.   Saez, E, Zucman, G. *The Triumph of Injustice: How the Rich Dodge Taxes and How to Make Them Pay*. New York. *W. W. Norton & Company*, 2019, p. 42.
5.   Garfield, R, Rudowitz, R, Damico, A. Understanding the intersection of Medicaid and work. *Kaiser Family Foundation*, January 5, 2018.
6.   Blumenthal, D. How the new U. S. tax plan will affect health care. *Harvard Business Review*, December 19, 2017.
7.   Abramsky, S. Trump administration wants to redefine the poverty line, shrinking public aid. *Truthout*, June 20, 2019.
8.   Lawson, A. Trump's budget calls for $1.8 trillion in cuts to earned benefits. *Social Security Works*, February 12, 2018.
9.   Jan, T, Dewey, C, Goldstein, A et al. Trump wants to overhaul America's safety net with giant cuts to housing, food stamps, and health care. *The Washington Post*, February 12, 2018.
10. Clemente, F. Under cover of Kavanaugh, Republicans passed huge tax cuts for the wealthy. *The Progressive Populist*, November 1, 2018.
11. Corporations paid 11.3 percent tax rates last year, a steep drop under Trump. *The Washington Post*, December 17, 2019, A17.
12. Pear, R. Congress warns against Medicaid cuts: 'You just wait for the firestorm.' *New York Times*, March 12, 2019.
13. Potter, W. Trump's greedy 2019 budget goes nuclear on Medicare and Medicaid. *Common Dreams*, March 13, 2019.
14. Kuttner, R. Conservatives mugged by reality. *The American Prospect*, July/August 2014, p. 5.
15. Rau, J. In the end, even the middle class would feel GOP cuts in nursing home care. *Kaiser Health News*, June 26, 2017.
16. Johnson J. A handful of billionaire families grab nation's wealth for themselves, new report details how dynasties rig U.S. economy. *Common Dreams*, October 30, 2018.
17. Ingraham, C. The richest 1 percent now owns more of the country's wealth than at any time in the past 50 years. *The Washington Post*, December 6, 2017.

18. Reich, R., as quoted by Queally, J. Even the 1% know they aren't paying their fair share: New poll shows 60 % of millionaires support Warren's ultra-wealth tax. *Common Dreams*, June 12, 2019.

19. Ibid #14.

20. Wilper, AP, Woolhandler, S, Lasser, K et al. Health insurance and mortality in U. S. adults. *American Journal of Public Health*, 99 (12): 2289-2295, 2009.

21. Sachs, J. America's health is declining and corporations are stoking the crisis. *CNN*, December 17, 2017.

22. Ibid # 4, p. xiii.

23. Galewitz, P. Medicaid covers all that? It's the backstop of America's ailing health system. *Kaiser Health News*, September 25, 2017.

24.. Bernstein, J, Katch, H. Trump administration's under-the-radar attack on Medicaid is gaining speed. *The Washington Post*, March 6, 2018.

25. Sommers, BD, Goldman, AL, Blendon, RJ et al. Medicaid work requirements—Results from the first year in Arkansas. *New England Journal of Medicine*, June 19, 2019.

26. Twain, M. As quoted in Budd, LJ (ed), Mark Twain: *Collected Tales, Sketches, Speeches, & Essays,* 1852-1890. New York. *The Library of America*, 1992, p. 289.

27. Corbett, J. Instead of death and destruction, poor people's moral budget shows what it looks like to 'invest in life.' *Common Dreams*, June 17, 2019.

PART III

WHAT CAN BE DONE?

The way we treat our children in the dawn of their lives, and the way we treat our elderly in the twilight of their lives, is a measure of the quality of a nation.

—Hubert Humphrey, Jr., Vice President
of the United States from 1965 to 1969

Health care is for people, not for profit. We don't need more reform of the insurance market. Insurance and markets are problems, not the solution. We need a health care system that cares for every American in every community.

—Michael Fine, M.D., leader of a population-based primary care
and public health collaboration in Central Falls, Rhode Island,
and author of *Health Care Revolt: How to Organize,
Build a Health Care System, and Resuscitate
Democracy —All at the Same Time.*

CHAPTER 10

FINANCING REFORM

Having seen in Chapter 3 of Part I the increasingly unaffordable costs for seniors needing long-term care, followed by Part II chapters describing how we got here, it is now time to consider how we can extricate ourselves from this unacceptable and unsustainable place. Recall some markers from those chapters:

- Trump's budget cuts of Social Security, Medicare and Medicaid will further decimate what safety net seniors and disabled Americans still have.
- Costs of long-term care for one person are often approaching $100,000 a year whether at home, nursing home, or assisted living facilities.
- More than two of five underinsured U. S. adults cannot afford to seek needed care.
- Because of the lack of a national policy for the increasing needs of our aging population for LTC, many individuals and families exhaust their financial resources in caring for their family members.
- Private long-term care insurance is disappearing, Medicare does not cover LTC, and Medicaid coverage is increasingly inadequate.
- Oversight of LTC is inadequate so that unacceptable quality of care is common, especially in for-profit facilities.
- There is a serious shortage of caregivers for LTC whether for home care, nursing home, or assisted living, largely due to their poverty level wages.

This chapter has two goals: (1) to consider various options for financing reform, including the case for and against Medicare for All; and (2) to describe the political landscape that will determine whether or not we can achieve real reform.

Financing Options for U. S. Health Care

The question front and center today is how to provide universal coverage for health care for all U.S. residents, everybody in, nobody out. Answering that question requires answers to these questions:

- Is health care a right, or a privilege based on ability to pay?
- Should health care services be not-for-profit or for-profit as just another commodity to be bought and sold in an unfettered marketplace?
- Who is our health care system for—patients and their families or corporate stakeholders in the medical-industrial complex?

Because these basic questions are still unanswered, it comes as no surprise that the current political debate reflects powerful corporate interests favoring the status quo and opposing answers in the public interest.

Many politicians on both sides of the aisle are arguing for incremental change, not as they see it, the more "radical" change they claim is represented by Medicare for All—single-payer national health insurance (NHI). The debate is sorting out into three warring camps—those wanting to build on the ACA, Republicans trying to devise their own "plan," and more progressive Democrats supporting single-payer NHI. Here are the three major reform alternatives.

1. Defending and Building on the Affordable Care Act (ACA)

Some Democrats in the House of Representatives are now proposing incremental options that can easily be confused with Medicare for All. The quite deceptively named Medicare for America, co-sponsored by Rosa DeLauro (D-CT) and Jan Schakowski (D-IL), would retain the private health insurance industry and employer-sponsored insurance, and enroll new enrollees under a new Medicare Part E plan. While it would upgrade benefits, it would charge premiums, require co-payments and deductibles capped at $3,500. As with Medicare Advantage, we can expect that insurers will inflate taxpayers' costs by cherry-picking healthier patients, enacting network restrictions, and avoiding sicker patients. [1]

Different incremental proposals are being supported by other Democrats in the House. These include Medicare Extra for All, proposed by the Center for American Progress, a liberal think tank, that would allow those covered by private insurance to continue it if they preferred [2]; a Medicare Public Option which could be available on the ACA's exchanges [3]; and a Medicare buy-in plan for adults between ages 50 and 64. [4]

None of these faux "Medicare for All" plans could ever get to universal coverage or achieve the kind of cost containment so urgently needed. This is because they sacrifice most of the price controls and administrative savings gained under single-payer plans.

Defenders of the ACA and other incremental proposals appear to be motivated to avoid the wrath of the private health insurance industry, as was done in the lead-up battle to the ACA in 2009. Aside from looking in the rear-view mirror for "reform" ideas, they also seem to disregard the actual track record of the ACA since it was enacted nine years ago:

- The ACA has failed to contain costs or improve the quality of care.
- ACA insurers have limited patients' choice and access to care through restrictive and changing networks.
- Premiums have gone up as profiteering by private insurers continues.
- The rolls of the uninsured and underinsured are climbing.[5]
- Sky-high deductibles are breaking the employer-sponsored health insurance system. [6]
- Middle-age Americans are now much more likely to die of heart disease than they were in 2010, when the ACA was enacted. [7]
- Many rural Americans struggle with financial insecurity and access to care. [8]

2. The GOP "plan"

This is really a non-plan promoting a number of ideas that support the current marketplace and promise to somehow improve health care with full choice of competing health plans. House Republicans came up with a 37-page white paper in June 2016 called *A Better Way* that brought forward such discredited features as consumer-directed health care, health savings accounts, high risk pools, selling insurance across state lines, and state waivers and block grants to reduce federal responsibility for Medicaid. It encouraged further privatization of Medicare, and favored "premium support" vouchers giving more control to private insurers. All of these provisions would shift more costs to patients, increase overall costs of health care, and reduce government oversight of corporate stakeholders. [9]

As we know, this "plan" went nowhere in the 2017 Congress, has proved to be an embarrassment to the GOP since then, and has not yet led to a revised, credible GOP plan. Trump tells us that he will introduce a "great plan" sometime soon, but Republicans in Congress are already leaning away from bringing up health care again.

In the absence of a real health care plan, the GOP continues to sabotage the ACA in every way they can, while hoping to skirt by the health care issue in the 2020 election cycle with disinformation and a relentless attack of Medicare for All as a "socialist" plot. The GOP also supports the advantages of "keeping your private insurance if you prefer," (most of which is employer-based), thereby disregarding the increasing cost and volatility of that coverage and the fact that it favors higher-income people over lower-income people.

3. Medicare for All—Single-Payer National Health Insurance (NHI)

There are two single-payer bills now being debated in Congress: S-1129 in the Senate, sponsored by Senator Bernie Sanders, and H. R. 1384 with Rep. Pramila Jayapal (D-WA) and Rep. Debbie Dingell (D-MI) as co-sponsors.

Expanded and Improved Medicare for All, as described in H.R. 1384, will bring:

- "A new system of national health insurance (NHI) based on medical need, not ability to pay, based on the principle that health care is not a privilege but a human right, with equity for all U. S. residents.
- Universal access to health care for all U. S. residents, with full choice of providers and hospitals anywhere in the country without any restrictive networks.
- Coverage of all medically necessary care, including outpatient and inpatient services, dental and vision care, prescription drugs, reproductive health, mental health, *and long-term care.*
- No cost-sharing such as copays and deductibles at the point of care; no more pre-authorizations or other restrictions now imposed by private insurers.
- Pharmaceutical reform, including independent and rigorous evaluation of the efficacy and safety of medications.
- Establishment of a national scientific body, free from political interference, to evaluate and make recommendations for effective treatments.

- Administrative simplification with efficiencies and cost containment through large-scale cost controls, including negotiated fee schedules, global budgeting of individual hospitals and other facilities, and bulk purchasing of drugs and medical devices.
- Elimination of employer-sponsored health insurance and the private health insurance industry, its large administrative overhead and profiteering converted to cost savings that enable universal coverage through a not-for-profit single-payer financing system.
- Improved quality of care and outcomes for both individuals and populations due to universal access to care.
- Shared risk for the costs of illness and accidents across the entire population of 326 million." [10]

The two single-payer bills are quite different, with the House bill much better in terms of coverage and other provisions. Senate bill 1129 has these problems:

- "It retains for-profit, investor ownership of facilities without global budgets.
- It maintains current Medicare payment models, resulting in higher costs.
- It does not cover long-term care services except by preserving Medicaid for that purpose, nor does it provide coverage for people with disabilities.
- It includes co-pays for prescription drugs, with a cap of $200 per year for each person enrolled in the program." [11]

There is only one way to accomplish universal coverage in a way that patients, families and taxpayers can afford—single-payer Medicare for All—H. R. 1384, which received hearings in the House in 2019. This bill, when enacted, will bring affordable, comprehensive health care to all U. S. residents, based on medical need, not ability to pay, and on the principle that health care is not a privilege, but a human right. All U. S. residents will have full choice of physician, other health professionals, hospitals and other facilities. Medicare for All will provide, for the first time, coverage for long-term care and supports.

We can afford Medicare for All through huge savings by eliminating the administrative waste, excess bureaucracy, and profiteering of our multi-payer financing system, together with progressive taxes whereby 95 percent of Americans will pay less than they do now for private health insurance and health care.

An excellent study by the Political Economy Research Institute (PERI) at the University of Massachusetts-Amherst projects that single-payer Medicare for All will save the U. S. $5.1 trillion over a decade through savings from our market-based, multi-payer system. Middle-class Americans will see savings up to 14 percent, while high-income Americans will have only a small increase in their spending on health care. (Figure 10.1) [12]

FIGURE 10.1

PERCENT CHANGE IN HEALTH CARE SPENDING UNDER MEDICARE FOR ALL BY INCOME LEVEL AND INSURANCE STATUS, 2016

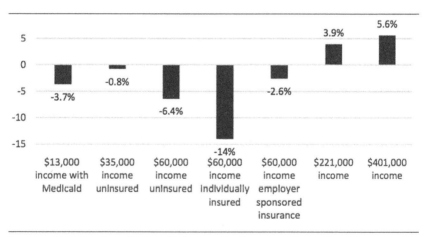

Sources: 2016 American Community Survey, the Consumer Expenditure Survey, and others.

Table 10.1 compares the outcomes of the three main alternatives for financing reform.[13]

TABLE 10.1

COMPARISON OF THREE
REFORM ALTERNATIVES

	ACA	*GOP*	*NHI*
Access	Restricted	Restricted	Unrestricted
Choice	Restricted	Restricted	Unrestricted
Cost containment	No	No	Yes
Quality of care	Unimproved	Unimproved	Improved
Bureaucracy	Increased	Increased	Much reduced
Universal coverage	Never	Never	Immediately
Accountability	Limited	Limited	Yes
Sustainability	No	No	Yes

Source: Geyman, J. *Crisis in U. S. Health Care: Corporate Power vs. the Common Good.* Friday Harbor, WA. *Copernicus Healthcare*, 2017, p. 305.

Public Interest vs. Corporate Power and Profits: Who Will Prevail?

National polls show wide and growing public support for single-payer Medicare for All, including 70 percent of all Americans, 85 percent of Democrats and 52 percent of Republicans. [14] Polls also find strong support for other parts of a progressive agenda—90 percent favor Medicare negotiating drug prices, two-thirds support expansion of Social Security, and three-quarters of voters believe that the tax system favors the rich and has too many loopholes, and a strong majority of voters favor doubling the minimal wage to $15 an hour. [15]

1. Support for the Public Interest

There are already 125 co-sponsors of H. R. 1384 in the House as momentum grows for further support in the Democratic caucus. Democrat 2020 presidential candidates are split on Medicare for All, some with strong support, others calling for incremental steps building on the ACA. [16]

Many groups support Medicare for All, including health professionals, who will welcome being relieved of the burden of dealing with billing through the multi-payer bureaucracy of Trumpcare. Employers will gain a healthier workforce as they no longer have to bear the increasing costs of covering their employees, and can better compete in a global market. Individuals will no longer be at risk for losing their health insurance when they change jobs. With the administrative simplicity of Medicare for All, taxpayers will pay less than they do now for health care and insurance, as government at both state and federal levels save money. Table 10.2 shows the winners and losers with Medicare for All. [17]

TABLE 10.2

WINNERS AND LOSERS UNDER SINGLE-PAYER MEDICARE FOR ALL

Winners	Losers
All Americans	Private health insurers
Physicians, other health professionals	Corporate middlemen
Hospitals	Corporate stakeholders
Employers	Privatized Medicare
Mental health care	Privatized Medicaid
Public health	Displaced workers
Federal and state governments	Lobbyists
Taxpayers	

Source: Geyman, J. *TrumpCare: Lies, Broken Promises, How It Is Failing and What Should Be Done. Copernicus Healthcare*, Friday Harbor, WA, 2018, p.246.

In advance of the House Budget Committee's first hearing, May 22, 2019, on Medicare for All, 209 economists sent an open letter to members of Congress, stating that:

> *As economists, we understand that a single-payer Medicare for All health insurance system for the U. S. can finance good-quality care for all U.S. residents as a basic right while still significantly reducing overall health care spending relative to the current exorbitant and wasteful system. Health care is not a service that follows standard market rules. It should therefor be provided as a public good. . . . The time is now to create a universal, single-payer Medicare for All health care system in the United States.* [18]

2. Support for Corporate Power and Profits

A large coalition of powerful corporate stakeholders, together with their lobbyists, are circling the wagons once again to defeat real health care reform—single-payer NHI—the only alternative that can bring universal coverage. Leading lobbyists for the pharmaceutical, insurance and hospital industries have formed the Partnership for America's Health Care Future to discredit and spread lies about Medicare for All. The AMA joined this coalition, against the efforts by the American Medical Students Association, representing future physicians of America, who strongly support Medicare for All. [19]

Wendell Potter, former insider at the health insurer Cigna, whom we met in the last chapter, analyzes the propaganda campaign by the private health insurance industry as spreading fear, uncertainty, and doubt (FUD). He notes these four specific examples:

"• FUD: We can't afford Medicare for All. TRUTH: We can't afford the status quo.
• FUD: Medicare for All will be too disruptive. TRUTH: Insurers and employers have been disrupting Americans for years to protect profits.

- FUD: Americans don't want "one-size-fits-all" health care. They want choice.
  TRUTH: It is not the choice of health insurance plans that Americans want, it is choice of doctors and hospitals.
- FUD: Americans who have employer-sponsored health insurance love it and don't want anything to replace it.
  TRUTH: The truth is that Americans are paying more and more every year for their employer-sponsored coverage and getting less and less value for the money they and their employers are spending for it." [20]

No surprise, given this assault on the truth, that confusion among the electorate is an ongoing problem, amplified by the efforts of the opposition of corporate stakeholders in the status quo. A multimillion-dollar ad campaign against Medicare for All has been launched by a GOP outside group aligned with Senate Majority Leader Mitch McConnell (R-KY). [21] The tentacles of opposition efforts are also bipartisan, especially involving campaign contributions targeting key Democrats. Rep. Cheri Bustos (D-IL), the new chair of the Democratic Congressional Campaign Committee (DCCC), is a good example of this. She is the favorite best friend of the health insurance industry, will have everything to do with the Democrats' 2020 platform, and already spreads fear that the costs of Medicare for All would be "scary." [22]

Opponents of Medicare for All often trot out the scare that it will be too disruptive to those with private employer-based health insurance. They avoid telling us, however, how volatile that coverage is, and that more U. S. workers are voluntarily leaving their jobs now than at any time since the quit rate has been recorded. A national survey by Mercer, a global HR consulting firm, found that more than 15 percent of employees voluntarily left their jobs in 2018. Figure 10.2 shows total employee quits since 2010, now approaching 40 million people a year. [23] All of these people lose their health insurance.

FIGURE 10.2

TOTAL EMPLOYEE QUITS HAVE RISEN EVERY YEAR SINCE 2010

The numbers below represent the total number of employee quits per year, in millions. Quits in 2018 are on track to exceed 40 million.

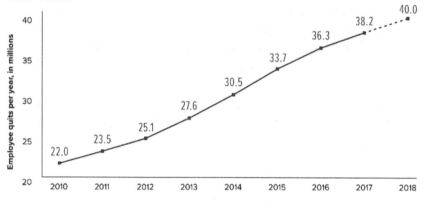

Source: U.S. Bureau of Labor Statistics

A recent study found that people insured in the private individual health insurance market tend to avoid switching plans because of inertia, the hassle of switching, and wanting to keep their choice of physicians and hospitals (typically not their choice of insurer). These reasons can lead them to pay up to $282 a month for continuing with that insurer! [24] Dr. Don McCanne, family physician of long experience and health policy expert, suggests that we arm ourselves with this additional question when considering our three main financing options:

> *Would you give up the insurance you now have if the new public plan was guaranteed for life, always providing you with your choice of physicians and hospitals, providing all essential benefits including mental health and long-term care, had no out-of-pocket costs whenever accessing health care, and was paid for by taxes that you could afford based on your ability to pay instead of being based on the high costs of care?* [25]

3. Who will prevail?

Clarifying the back and forth debate over single-payer NHI, Drs. Woolhandler and Himmelstein, health policy experts and co-founders of Physicians for a National Health Program in the late 1980s, bring us this important insight:

> *Halfway measures are politically attractive but economically unworkable. The $11,559 per capita that the United States spends on health care could provide high-quality care for all or it can continue to fund a vast health-managerial apparatus—it cannot do both.* [26]

Single-payer Medicare for All has become a political football even within leadership of the Democratic Party. House Speaker Rep. Nancy Pelosi (D-CA) has approved committee hearings for H. R. 1384, but wants to incrementally build on the ACA as her own legacy. Tom Perez, as chair of the Democratic National Committee (DNC) with much to say about the Party's 2020 platform, wants to empower the grassroots electorate, but remains a centrist unwilling to lead toward Medicare for All despite strong public polling for it. This turmoil within the Democratic establishment prompted Ronald Brownstein to observe in his article in *The Atlantic:*

> *How the debate turns out [over whether to retain the existing employer-based health insurance system or replace it completely by a single-payer financing structure] will gauge the new power among Democrats, as the party still envisions itself as the voice of the struggling, but represents a growing number of the comfortable.* [27]

Conclusion

As this debate unfolds, we need to remember that by doing nothing and keeping the status quo, more than 36 million people will be uninsured in 2027 as health care costs soar to almost $6 trillion. [28] Insurance deductibles and drug prices will keep going up, and the mortality gap between the rich and poor will widen.[29] The status quo is neither acceptable nor sustainable. We can do better than that, but only if we build a responsive government role, which Democrats should support.

We are at a crossroads on this issue, and could well learn from this helpful insight by Jacob Hacker and Paul Pierson, professors of political science at Yale University and the University of California Berkeley, respectively and authors of the important 2016 book, *American Amnesia: How the War on Government Led Us to Forget What Made America Prosper*:

> *It takes government—a lot of government—for advanced societies to flourish. But Americans have never been good at acknowledging government's necessary role in supporting both freedom and prosperity . . .The United States got rich because it got government more or less right. We suffer, in short from a kind of mass historical forgetting, a distinctively 'American Amnesia.'* [30]

So what can we expect to happen on this critical issue? This summary view from *Public Citizen* is spot-on:

> *We will be able to pass Medicare for All only by continuing to build grassroots support and taking on entrenched health care interests. The people power on this issue continues to intensify as Americans feel the pain of a health care system that is focused more on profit than it is on providing health care. Polls show that Americans are hungry for bold, systematic transformation of the system. While it's true that those who profit from the current system will put everything they have behind hindering reform, it is impossible to override the moral imperative that everyone in the U. S. deserves access to health care. The American people won't stop pushing for significant change. The question is not if we will win, it is when.* [31]

References

1. Woolhandler, S, Himmelstein, DU. Medicare for All and its rivals: New offshoots of old health policy roots. *Annals of Internal Medicine*, April 2. 2019.
2. CAP Health Policy Team. Medicare Extra for All. *Center for American Progress*, February 22, 2018.
3. Ibid # 1.
4. Kirzinger, A, Munana, C, Brodie, M. KFF Health Tracking Poll—January 2019: The public on next steps for the ACA and proposals to expand coverage. *Kaiser Family Foundation*, January 23, 2019.
5. Cohen, RA, Terllizzi, EP, Martinez, ME. Health insurance coverage: Early release of estimates from the National Health Interview Survey, 2018. U.S. Department of Health and Human Services, Centers for Disease Control and Prevention, National Center for Health Statistics, May 2019.
6. Levey, NN. Health insurance deductibles soar, leaving Americans with unaffordable bills. *Los Angeles Times*, May 2, 2019.
7. McKay, B. Heart disease roars back. *Wall Street Journal*, June 22-23, 2019: A1.
8. Neel, J, Neighmond, P. Poll: Many rural Americans struggle with financial insecurity, access to health care. *NPR Newscast*, May 21, 2019.
9. Rovner, J. House Republicans unveil long-awaited plan to replace health law. *Kaiser Health News*, June 22, 2016.
10. Geyman, J. *Common Sense: The Case For and Against Medicare for All: Leading Issue in the 2020 Elections*. Friday Harbor, WA, *Copernicus Healthcare*, May 2019, pp. 3-4.
11. Geyman, J. *Struggling and Dying Under Trumpcare: How We Can Fix This Fiasco*. Friday Harbor, WA. *Copernicus Healthcare*, 2019, p, 172.
12. Pollin, R, Heintz, J, Arno, P et al. *In-Depth Analysis by Team of UMass Amherst Economists Shows Viability of Medicare for All*. Amherst, MA, November 30, 2018.
13. Geyman, J. *Crisis in U. S. Health Care: Corporate Power vs. the Common Good*. Friday Harbor, WA. *Copernicus Healthcare*, 2017, p. 305.
14. Conley, J. New analysis shows why Democrats are wrong to fear bold embrace of Medicare for All. *Common Dreams*, January 14, 2019.
15. Weissman, R. Progressive policies are popular politics. *Public Citizen*, May/June 2019, p. 3.
16. Armour, S. Peril awaits parties on health care. *Wall Street Journal*, June 3, 2019: A4.

17. Geyman, J. *Trumpcare: Lies, Broken Promises, How It Is Failing, and What Must Be Done.* Friday Harbor, WA. *Copernicus Healthcare*, 2018, p. 246.
18. Johnson, J. 'It's a sure winner—except for the profiteers': 200+ economists send letter to Congress endorsing Medicare for All. *Common Dreams*, May 21, 2019.
19. Michels, J, Cox, W, Siddula, A et al. Why we're fighting the American Medical Association. *The Guardian*, June 6, 2019.
20. Potter, W. I used to be a propagandist for insurance companies. Learn the four truths the insurance industry doesn't want Americans to see. *Tarbell*, April 30, 2019.
21. Sullivan, P. McConnell-aligned group launches $4M ad campaign against Medicare for All. *The Hill*, June 20, 2019.
22. Potter, W. Democrats on the take: New DCCC chair is a best friend of health insurers. *Tarbell*, March 15, 2019.
23. Maurer, R. Why are workers quitting their jobs in record numbers? SHRM, December 12, 2018.
24. Ryan, C, Dowd, B. Sources of inertia in health plan choice in the individual health insurance market. 8th Conference of the American Society of Health Economists, June 23-26, 2019.
25. McCanne, D. Commentary on reference 23. Quote of the Day. June 28, 2019. don@mccanne.org.
26. Woolhandler, S, Himmelstein, DU. Single-payer reform—"Medicare for All". *JAMA* on line, May 31, 2019.
27. Brownstein, R. The coming Democratic drama over Medicare for All. *The Atlantic*, January 31, 2019.
28. Sisko, AM, Keehan, SP, Poisal, JA et al. National health expenditure projections, 2018-2027: economic and demographic trends drive spending and enrollment growth. *Health Affairs (Millwood)* 38(10): 377, 2019.
29. Ibid # 1.
30. Hacker, JS, Pierson, P. *American Amnesia: How the War on Government Led Us to Forget What Made America Prosper.* New York. *Simon & Schuster*, 2016, pp. 1-2.
31. *The Case for Medicare for All. Public Citizen.* Washington, DC, February 4, 2019.

CHAPTER 11

RE-VALUING LONG-TERM CARE AND CAREGIVERS

As we saw in Chapter 7, long-term care has been undervalued across the board for many years. Following up on this major problem, this chapter has three goals:

(1) to briefly summarize the dimensions of the critical current and future shortage of long-term caregivers; (2) to discuss seven approaches to address this shortage; and (3) to consider what is being done at federal and state levels to address this growing crisis.

Magnitude of the Problem

To begin with, we have to recognize that the majority of home health care is carried out on an informal and unpaid basis by family members caring for other family members. In 2011, more than 90 percent of elders receiving help with activities of daily living (ADLs) received some informal care, and about two-thirds received *only* informal care. Informal family caregivers accounted for 75 to 80 percent of total care hours in that year. [1] A 2014 report from the Alzheimer's Association found that 15 million family members provided over 17 *billion* hours of unpaid care to those with Alzheimer's disease and other dementias in 2013, more than 1,000 hours of care per caregiver. [2]

While informal family caregiving is at the heart of the goal of enabling elders to age in place despite increasing disabilities, there are limits to that care, as we saw in Chapter 2, that make formal, non-family long-term caregivers extremely important. However, the current and future shortage of long-term caregivers is a serious, multifaceted problem.

Although one in seven low-wage women is a home care aide, they have a difficult time in life. Home care workers are devalued, underpaid, mostly low-income women with families of their own, and struggling to make ends meet. Most live in poverty, their work is hard and at high-risk for injury, but most labor on without paid sick leave. There is a high turnover rate among caregivers, thereby decreasing quality of their care because of discontinuity.

To clarify the direct care workforce, Table 11.1 lists the occupational titles and industry classifications of home care workers. [3] Nursing assistants perform the same work as Home Health Aides (HHAs), but are usually employed in nursing homes.

TABLE 11.1

TITLES AND JOB DESCRIPTIONS OF HOME CARE WORKERS

TITLE	OTHER TITLES	JOB DESCRIPTION
Personal Care Aides (SOC 39-9021)	Personal Care Attendant, Personal Assistant, Direct Support Professional (for people with intellectual and developmental disabilities); also includes Independent Providers (employed directly by consumers)	In addition to assisting with activities of daily living (ADLs), personal care aides often help with housekeeping, chores, meal preparation, and medication management. They also help individuals go to work and remain engaged in their communities, and they advise on nutrition, household maintenance, and other activities.
Home Health Aides (SOC 31-1011)	Home Hospice Aide, Home Health Attendant	In addition to assisting with ADLs, home health aides also perform clinical tasks such as wound care, blood pressure readings, and range-of-motion exercises. Their work is supervised by licensed nurses or therapists.
Nursing Assistants (SOC 31-1014)	Certified Nursing Assistant, Certified Nursing Aide, Nursing Attendant, Nursing Aide, Nursing Care Attendant	In most states, nursing assistant credentials are portable to home- and community-based settings. In the context of home care, nursing assistants perform the same work as home health aides.

Source: *U. S. Home Care Workers. Key Facts.* Paraprofessional Healthcare Institute (PHI) National, 2019

Because of the increasing demand for non-medical in-home support, the home care workforce has more than doubled over the last 10 years. Personal care aides have accounted for three-quarters of that growth. (Figure 11.1) But that will still fall far short of future needs. The Bureau of Labor Statistics (BLS) projects that 8.2 million direct care jobs will need to be filled by 2028 due to high demand and high turnover within that workforce. BLS also tells us that the direct care workforce will be the fastest growing occupation in the country. [4]

FIGURE 11.1

HOMECARE WORKER EMPLOYMENT BY OCCUPATION, 2008 TO 2018

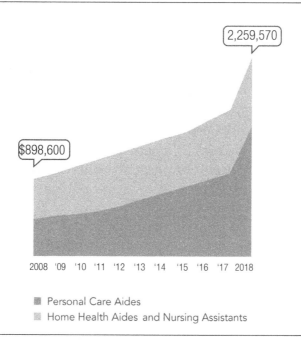

Source: *U. S. Home Care Workers. Key Facts.* Paraprofessional Healthcare Institute (PHI) National, 2019

These two caregiver stories illustrate the magnitude and breadth of this problem. [5]

Kimberly Weems, Atlanta, GA

I've been a home care worker for 14 years. I started off taking care of my blind uncle when I was young. I love helping others; I'm passionate about enabling seniors and people with disabilities to stay in their homes and communities.

Independence is one of the most important aspects of home care. My granddaughter was born with a disability, and I want her to be able to stay in her home with her family and receive the best care possible.

Despite all my years of experience, my pay has actually dropped over the years. I currently make just $8.50 an hour.

It's time to start paying home care workers a living wage, because quality jobs mean quality care.

Patricia Evans, Chicago, IL

When it comes to home care workers, you live in poverty. You work in poverty. You retire poor, hoping you will qualify for the services you have provided for so many years to others. Then, you die in poverty.

That's just not right. We make a real difference in peoples' lives. We're people of worth. We make a valuable contribution to society, and it's time that our paychecks reflected that.

Approaches to the Caregiver Shortage

Since the family caregiver shortage is so complicated and multifaceted, a broad range of approaches will be required to address this problem. These seven initiatives will go a long way towards that goal.

1. Raise wages

According to the U. S. Bureau of Labor Statistics, the median hourly wage for home care workers in 2018 was $11.52. With their unpredictable work hours, their typical annual earnings were $16,200, close to the federal poverty level. They often need two or more clients at a time, and one-half of the workforce turns over every year, mostly because they cannot afford to stay. Their real wages adjusted for inflation have risen only slightly over the last ten years. (Figure 11.2) and are lower than most other jobs. (Figure 11.3) As a result of their near-poverty wages, more than one half of home care workers receive some form of public assistance.[6]

FIGURE 11.2

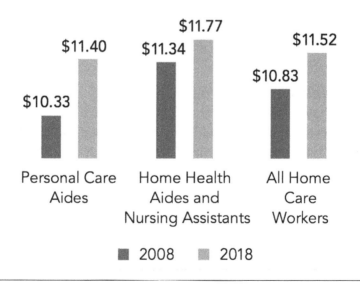

HOME CARE WORKER MEDIAN HOURLY WAGES ADJUSTED FOR INFLATION, 2008 TO 2018

Source: *Paying the Price: How Poverty Wages Undermine Home Care in America.* New York, NY. Paraprofessional Healthcare Institute National, 2019, p. 5.

FIGURE 11.3

WAGE CRUNCH FOR HOME CARE WORKERS

Hourly pretax pay for the aides and assistants who provide the majority of hands-on care for the elderly and people with disabilities is lower than that of many jobs. The median hourly wage for all U.S. workers is $18.12.

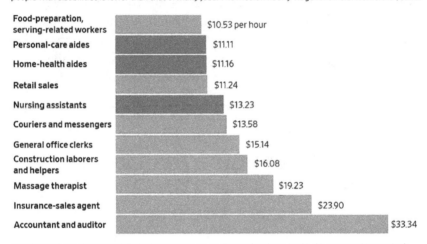

Food-preparation, serving-related workers	$10.53 per hour
Personal-care aides	$11.11
Home-health aides	$11.16
Retail sales	$11.24
Nursing assistants	$13.23
Couriers and messengers	$13.58
General office clerks	$15.14
Construction laborers and helpers	$16.08
Massage therapist	$19.23
Insurance-sales agent	$23.90
Accountant and auditor	$33.34

Note: Personal-care aides generally limited to providing non-medical services; home-health aides may provide some basic health-related services; nursing assistants listen to and record patient's health concerns and report information to nurses

Source: Bureau of Labor Statistics

2. Provide paid sick leave

Although seven states and the District of Columbia have passed laws that require paid family and medical leave, most home care workers cannot leave their jobs to care for an aging parent, cope with a difficult pregnancy, or bond with a child while still being paid. [7]

3. Provide health care coverage

Four in ten direct care workers have health insurance, mostly through Medicaid, but about 20 percent have no coverage. They have seen small gains in employer-based coverage, but that is limited by their often part-time work status. [8] The lack of health insurance is a big problem in their high-risk work, since they often are injured by having to lift and move much heavier patients without anyone else's help. Moreover, they are more likely to have chronic health conditions and be at higher risk for infection than the average U. S. worker. [9,10]

4. Increase public investment and funding

More than one-half of homecare workers already rely on some form of public benefits. But better wages, such as by adopting a $15.00 minimal hourly wage, could lift millions of poor families out of poverty while cutting expenditures for such public support programs as Medicaid. Better wages could also bring a multiplier effect by enabling their families to spend their increased wages on goods and services in their communities. Studies have estimated that every $1.00 an-hour increase in compensation for low-wage workers leads to $1.20 increase in economic activity as they spend their earnings on basic necessities of life. [11]

5. Increase training

Although many states have some requirements for home health aides (HHAs) who have responsibility for some medical care, most states have little or no requirements for personal care assistants (PCAs). States tend to rely on home care agencies to provide orientation and training for PCAs, but in fact most provide little or none. [12]

A recent study by the Paraprofessional Healthcare Institute (PHI) has updated the current level of training across the country for PCAs, with these findings:

- "14 states have consistent training requirements for all agency-employed PCAs, while 7 states do not regulate training for PCAs at all. The other 29 states and the District of Columbia have varying requirements for agency-employed PCAs, depending whether they work in specific Medicaid programs or for private-pay home care agencies.

- 26 states require a minimum number of training hours for PCAs in at least one set of training requirements, including 15 states and the District of Columbia that require 40 or more hours of training.
- 34 states and the District of Columbia require PCAs to complete a competency assessment after training in at least one set of training regulations.
- 17 states regulate instruction methods in at least one set of regulations, including 11 states and the District of Columbia that require trainers to use a state-sponsored curriculum or curriculum outline." [13]

Increased training for home care workers has been shown to improve care, patient and family satisfaction, and also to reduce burnout and turnover of caregivers. [14] The Paraprofessional Healthcare Institute has adopted this model curriculum for home care workers:

- "Introduction to the direct care setting
- Professionalism and teamwork
- Infection control
- Body mechanics
- Body systems and common diseases
- Working with elders
- Respecting differences
- Communication skills
- Supporting consumers safely at home
- Ambulating and making a bed
- Supporting patient dignity while providing care
- Bathing and personal care
- Working with Alzheimer's disease patients
- Dressing and toileting
- Working with an independent adult with physical disabilities
- Eating
- Depression, mental illness, abuse and neglect
- Consumer and worker rights
- Managing time and managing stress." [15]

6. Offer opportunities for career advancement

Despite their importance, direct caregivers are still held back as an undervalued occupation with low wages, inadequate benefits, and little or no opportunity for advancement. The Obama administration attempted to address this problem in 2013 by declaring that, starting in 2015, personal care workers should no longer be classified as companions and should become eligible for minimum wage, overtime, and other benefits set by the Fair Labor Standards Act for non-exempt employees. According to a Home Care Final Rule issued by the U. S. Department of Labor in 2016, most home care workers must now be paid at least the federal minimum wage and overtime pay. [16]

In 2014, the Eldercare Workforce Alliance, a consortium of 31 organizations dedicated to caregiving for older adults, issued a consensus policy brief calling for the development of an Advanced Direct Care Worker position for federal long-term care programs. An expanded training program would target the need to fill caregiver gaps through these curricular areas:

- *Assistance with medical and nursing needs* (egs. catheter care, wound care, medication monitoring and administration, recognition of common medical symptoms and drug side effects.)
- *Providing health information and resources* (egs. health promotion, nutrition, proper dental care, prescribed exercises.)
- *Care coordination* (egs. communication skills, cultural competency, ethics of patient care.) [17]

7. Enact supportive immigrant policies

One million immigrants are employed in the direct care workforce in the U. S., as personal care aides, home health aides, or as nursing assistants. They continue to play a vital role in the nation's system of long-term care. [18]

Although more than one-quarter of home care workers were born outside the United States, 86 percent are U. S. citizens. Almost 90 percent of home care workers are women, 60 percent are people of color, their median age is 47, and one-half have completed no formal education beyond high school. Since employment in home care jobs has minimal legal and employer-based requirements for education, training, and experience, workers often find opportunities in home care when they would otherwise encounter educational, language, or discriminatory barriers [19]

Trumps's zero-tolerance policies on immigration cause cruel and documented harm to applicants for asylum on the southern border, with detention camps far above occupancy levels and with hundreds of human beings forced to stand up 24-7 for many days awaiting processing.

Immigrant workers have, and will continue to play a major role in LTC, and are hardly taking jobs away from U. S. born Americans. Dr. Louise Aronson, geriatrician and professor of medicine at the University of California San Francisco, and author of the 2019 book, *Elderhood: Redefining Aging, Transforming Medicine, Reimagining Life*, makes this observation:

> *While there may be sectors of the economy in which undocumented workers take jobs from Americans, in twenty years of geriatrics, I had only met a handful of working- or lower-middle-class families who had been able to find an American willing to care for their aging relative for a salary they could afford. Even the upper and upper-middle classes, with enough money to pay the going rate or more, struggle to find caregivers. Often, when they do, they pay higher rates, most of which go to agencies, while the caregivers themselves—those people in whose hands a loved one's life and well-being are placed—still receive minimum wage.* [20]

New Directions Toward Dealing with the Caregiver Crisis

Although we still don't have a coherent national plan for addressing this increasing crisis in long-term care in this country, important progress is being made, even toward paying family member caregivers.

1. Examples charting new directions in long-term care.

- The home care workforce has more than doubled in size over the last ten years from almost 899,000 in 2008 to 2.3 million in 2018. [21]
- Long-term care is increasingly shifting from institutional locations, such as nursing homes, to home and community settings across the U. S. [22]
- About 500,000 direct care workers gained health insurance between 2010 and 2014, mostly due to Medicaid expansion under the ACA in 31 states and the District of Columbia. [23]
- One-half of the states now include personal care services in their Medicaid programs, including payment for LTC services by family members and friends. [24]
- The U. S. Department of Labor issued a new rule that extends minimum wage and overtime compensation to most home care workers. [25]
- About one-quarter of direct care workers have formed unions, whereby they can now negotiate wages and working conditions. [26]
- The Expanded and Improved Medicare for All bill in the House (H. R. 1384), when and if enacted, will provide funding for LTC services across the country for the first time.

2. Organizations that have led the way toward expanding and improving the direct care workforce:

- PHI. *The Paraprofessional Health Institute* was established more than 25 years ago, with the mission to transform eldercare and disability services. As the leading authority on the direct care workforce, it carries out ongoing monitoring and research targeting best practices and evidence-based policies that advance quality of care. [27]

- *The National Caregiver Support Program (NCSP)*, established in 2000 under the Administration for Community Living, provides grants to states and territories to fund various supports that help family and other informal caregivers care for older adults in their homes for as long as possible. The NCSP was reauthorized by Congress through the 2016 Reauthorization of the Older Americans Act. [28]

- *Universal Family Care*. This is the latest entrant to the national effort to expand and improve the direct care workforce. In 2019, the Study Panel of the non-partisan National Academy of Social Insurance (NASI) released an important new report, *Designing Universal Family Care*, which recommends policy options to state policy makers for early child care and education, long-term services and supports, and paid family and medical leave. [29] This organization creates a social insurance program providing affordable early child care, paid leave, assistance for people with disabilities, and elder care for people of all incomes. Enrollees will contribute small amounts from every paycheck from their first job on, then sign up for benefits when needed. [30]

3. Progress in a number of states and cities.

- *Cooperative Home Care Associates (CHCA)* is a work-er-owned cooperative employing more than 2,000 home care aides in New York City's low-income neighbor-hoods. By 2015, it had succeeded in raising their wages and benefits to more than $14.00 an hour, including paid leave and health coverage. Training has been upgraded, advancement opportunities are now in place, and the an-nual turnover rate has dropped to less than 15 percent, far below the industry average. [31]

- *Washington State's Long-Term Care Trust Act of 2019* is the nation's first public state-operated long-term care in-surance program. It will pay benefits of up to $36,500 for those needing assistance with ADLs. It will be funded by a payroll tax of 0.58 percent on employees, and be avail-able for a wide range of services. It is expected that this plan will cost a middle-income worker only about $300 a year. There will be a transitional delay—the state will start to collect the tax in 2022 and pay benefits from 2025 on. [32]

Conclusion

As is now obvious, we are way behind the curve in meeting the LTC needs of our aging population and still far short of the number of direct care workers needed in the U.S. Progress is being made, but there is a long way to go.

Dr. Henry Moss, whom we met in Chapter 5, puts the breadth of his training, research, and experience to envision the goal to train an army of direct care workers, mobilizing two-year colleges and other training facilities in this effort. He calls for some kind of federally directed or endorsed certification that would "affirm the value of the worker, make it easier to transfer between jobs and states, and ensure the integrity of federally-funded long-term care programs." And further, he leaves us with this challenge:

The 2030 crisis is forcing us, as a nation, to address this need for shared responsibility. The problem is bigger than any one person. Disability, dementia, and depression can afflict an older adult in any segment of society and inflict emotional distress in even the wealthiest.

If everyone recognizes the problem and wants a solution, obstacles associated with budgets and finance can be overcome. They were overcome when Medicare and Social Security were first developed. They were overcome in World War II. The crisis cannot be addressed without better pay and training for direct care workers and without providing round-the-clock care in a home setting. The crisis cannot be addressed without expanding nursing homes and special care units, and improving their staffing and conditions. The crisis cannot be addressed without providing financial support to family caregivers forced to leave the workforce to care for a loved one. [33]

References

1. Spillman, B, Wolff, J, Freedman, V et al. Informal Caregiving for Older Americans: An Analysis of the 2011 National Health and Aging Trends Study. Washington, DC U. S. Department of Health and Human Services, 2014.
2. Alzheimer's Association. Staying Safe. (Brochure). Chicago, IL, 2014.
3. U. S. Home Care Workers. Key Facts. Paraprofessional Healthcare Institute (PHI) National, September 2019, pp. 9-10.
4. Campbell, S. Personal communication. Paraprofessional Healthcare Institute National (PHI), November 7, 2019.
5. *Paying the Price: How Poverty Wages Undermine Home Care in America.* New York, NY. Paraprofessional Healthcare Institute National, 2015.
6. Ibid # 3, pp. 2, 5.
7. Ansberry, C. Caregivers do double duty to stay afloat. *Wall Street Journal,* October 29, 2018; A 17.

8. Poo, A, Veghte, B. The big, feminist policy idea America's families have been waiting for. *New York Times,* June 23, 2019.
9. McCaughey, D, McGhan, G, Kim, J et al. Workforce implications of injury among home health workers: Evidence from the Home Health Aide Survey. *The Gerontologist* 52 (4): 493-505, 2012.
10. Marquand, A. Too Sick to Care: Direct Care Workers, Medicaid Expansion, and the Coverage Gap. Bronx, NY. Paraprofessional Health Institute, 2015.
11. Cooper, D, Hall, D. Raising the federal minimum wage to $10.10 would give working families, and the overall economy, a much needed boost. *Economic Policy Institute,* Washington, DC, 2013.
12. Marquand, A, Chapman, S. The national landscape of personal care aide training standards. Health Workforce Research Center, San Francisco, CA, 2014.
13. Personal Care Aide Training Requirements. Paraprofessional Healthcare Institute (PHI), 2019.
14. *The role of training in improving the recruitment and retention of direct-care workers in long-term care.* New York, NY. Paraprofessional Healthcare Institute, 2005.
15. *Providing personal care services to elders and people with disabilities: A model curriculum for direct-care workers.* New York, NY. Paraprofessional Healthcare Institute, 2009.
16. *Paying Minimum Wages and Overtime to Home Care Workers: A Guide for Consumers and Their Families to the Fair Labor Standards Act,* 2016. U. S. Department of Labor.
17. Issue Brief. *Advanced Direct Care Worker: A role to improve quality and efficiency of care for older adults and strengthen career ladders for home care workers.* Washington, DC Eldercare Workforce Alliance, 2014.
18. Ibid # 3, p. 3.
19. Campbell, S. Immigration's effect on the direct care worker supply. *Aging Today,* January/February, 2018.
20. Aronson, L. *Elderhood: Redefining Aging, Transforming Medicine, Reimagining Life.* New York. *Bloomsbury Publishing,* 2019, p. 327.
21. Ibid # 3, p. 4.
22. Ibid # 3, p. 2.
23. Campbell, S. *Issue Brief. The Impact of the Affordable Care Act on Health Coverage for Direct Care Workers.* Paraprofessional Healthcare Institute, New York, NY, March 2017.
24. Moss, H. *The 2030 Caregiving Crisis: A Heavy Burden for Boomer Children.* Bronx, NY. 2015, p. 174.
25. Ibid # 19.
26. Ibid # 5, p. 14.

27. Ibid # 25, p. 7.
28. Ibid # 8.
29. Nonpartisan expert panel examines policy options to better support families and caregivers. National Academy of Social Insurance, June 24, 2019.
30. Ibid # 10.
31. Ibid # 5, p. 16.
32. Gleckman, H. What you need to know about Washington State's Public Long-Term Care Insurance Program. *Forbes*, May 15, 2019.
33. Ibid # 24 , p. 196.

CHAPTER 12

REIMAGINING THE FUTURE
OF LONG-TERM CARE

The U. S., in effect, has two health systems. One addresses disease, the science of what makes us sick; the other addresses illness, the human experience of being sick. Disease demands treatment, while illness calls out for care. . . . We must find the resources to elevate and compensate the dwindling ranks of home health workers. And we must build into the system support for the millions of family members whose determination and sacrifice sustain and enrich the lives of their loved ones. True health care must include care.

—Arthur Kleinman, M. D., professor of medical anthropology
and psychiatry at Harvard Medical School and author, most recently,
of *The Soul of Care: The Moral Education of a Husband and a Doctor.* [1]

Disability does not mean inability. It means adaptability.

—New York City Mayor Fiorello La Guardia, welcoming home
combat veterans from World War II in October, 1945

Now that we have seen the problems of our non-system for LTC that serves corporate stakeholders more than patients and families, it is time to imagine a better future for long-term care in this country. We should have learned the lessons that will help to rebuild a system that meets the critical and increasing needs of our aging society.

We have three goals for this final chapter: (1) to consider societal views about aging and disabilities; (2) to outline the characteristics of an expanded and improved system for LTC; and (3) to briefly discuss issues around palliative care when cure is no longer possible, together with person-centered end-of-life care.

1. Societal Views of Aging and Disability

Just as we have an undervalued system for LTC in the U. S., our society also has many negative attitudes toward aging itself, people with disabilities, and those who become frail and/or develop dementia. Negative stereotypes abound in our youth-oriented culture, with ageism even more common than sexism and racism. Old people tend to become more invisible as they age. Recall Dr. Aronson's revised human life cycle with its expected phases of decreasing independence and increasing dependence during later elderhood. (Figure 8.1, page 107) [2]

We have yet to come to grips with the extended longevity that the 20th century brought us. Dr. Laura Carstensen, professor of psychology and director of the Stanford Center of Longevity, brings us this important insight:

> *It's time to get serious about a major redesign of life. Thirty years were added to average life expectancy in the 20th century, and rather than imagine the scores of ways we could use these years to improve quality of life, we tacked them all on at the end. Only old age got longer. . . Long lives are not the problem. The problem is living in cultures designed for lives half as long as the lives we have.* [3]

The devaluation of LTC, with its low funding priority, reflects our society that gives short shrift to the elderly, quite different from its high attention to childhood and adulthood. Even many physicians reflect attitudes of ageism as they approach older patients. Here is just one example:

> *A 97-year-old man goes to his doctor with a painful left knee, without any history of a fall or other trauma. After examining the knee, the doctor dismissively says: "Hey, the knee is 97 years old, what do you expect?" The patient replies: But my right knee is 97 and doesn't hurt a bit!* [1]

Ernest Hemingway described bankruptcy happening in one of two ways—slowly and then all at once. There is a parallel with aging. Aging also happens in two ways, slowly and then all at once. The slow way to age is the familiar one; decades pass with little sense of internal change, middle age arrives with only a slight slowing down—a name lost, a lumbar ache, a sprinkling of white hairs and eye wrinkles. The fast way to age happens as a series of lurches: eyes occlude, hearing dwindles, a hand trembles where it didn't, a fall and a broken hip—the usual hale and hearty doctor's murmur in the yearly checkup, *"There are some signs here that concern me."* [5]

For most of us, the slow way is more likely, with decreasing independence and progressive disabilities, though often unpredictable. Dr. Aronson, as a geriatrician with long experience, whom we met in the last chapter, brings us these positive insights as to how she approaches patients as they age along their journeys:

> *"I have 5 priorities in assessing patients and helping them age well:*
> 1. *Focus on the whole person,*
> 2. *Emphasize fitness and prevention,*
> 3. *Ask "what are your goals and values; what makes you happy?",*
> 4. *Ask "what are your priorities?", and*
> 5. *Gain perspective by saying: "Let's figure out a way for you to keep doing the things that are important to you. Do you need new skills? Do you need to change your environment? Do you need to do a bit of both?"*[6]

Dr. Eric Larson, clinical professor of medicine at the University of Washington in Seattle, experienced geriatrician and co-author of the 2017 book, *Enlightened Aging: Building Resilience for a Long, Active Life,* promotes resilience as a way for his aging patients to adapt and grow stronger in the face of stress or adversity. Toward this goal, he finds these 3 interrelated steps useful:

1. *Proactivity:* Taking charge, in partnership with your health care providers, of your own health and happiness by preventing illness, managing chronic conditions, and getting care that's right for you—not too little and not too much;
2. *Acceptance:* Knowing change will come with age, which allows you to approach the future with equanimity and mindfulness—in large part by knowing your own values; and
3. *Three reservoirs:* Building reserves of well-being in three ways—mentally, physically, and socially—for the long, fulfilling road ahead. [7]

Many people in this country are now rejecting negative stereotypes about aging as they themselves age, especially within the baby boomer generation. Many say that they feel younger than they are, and hold to a positive view of their futures. [8] Perhaps surprisingly, some studies have shown that even disabled people often rate the quality of their lives higher than clinicians or the public do.[9] Dr. Tia Powell, author of *Dementia Reimagined: Building a Life of Joy and Dignity from Beginning to End,* observes that:

> *Disabled people frequently rate the quality of their lives higher than clinicians and the general public do. Living with a challenge, physical or cognitive, is consistent with a good life. Disabled people prove this every day. Our own growing disability is an unavoidable part of aging. We need to figure out how to find happiness within that reality, or we will not be happy. There is no other option.* [10]

Judy Heumann, co-founder and leader of the civil rights activist organization, Disabled in Action since 1970, as a young woman sued the Board of Education in New York City when she was denied her license to teach. She won and has long fought against stereotypes of people with disabilities this way:

> *It is not our disability that handicaps us; it is society that handicaps us . . . Disability only becomes a tragedy for us when society fails to provide the things we need to live our lives. It's a tragedy when we're discriminated against, kept out, treated as inferior.* [11]

Then there's the matter of how we should best view patients with advancing dementia. Drawing on the legendary work of Stephen Post, author of the 2000 book, *The Moral Challenge of Alzheimer Disease* and an activist in changing the culture of nursing homes to a stronger emphasis on quality of life, Dr. Powell further suggests:

> *Our society places too great a premium on cognition, and that is not the cardinal feature of a person. The capacity to feel emotions, to experience well-being or its absence, to respond to kindness and cruelty, all remain for the person with dementia, and are a better basis for respect than cognitive function. People with dementia should not be viewed as the sum of their losses, but rather as people with assets and liabilities, more like than unlike others.* [12]

Toward the Future: Improved Long-Term Care

In view of the problems of LTC described in earlier chapters, the goal of future long-term care should be to meet the expanding demands of our aging society. Since most people prefer home care as long as possible, without moving to an institutional setting, how can we gain a system where aging in place becomes the norm?

To do so, these 9 characteristics of new, improved LTC can accomplish that goal.

1. Public insurance coverage for patients regardless of age

Since we already know that private long-term care insurance is a relic of the past, that today's Medicare does not cover LTC, and that its costs are no longer affordable by so many needing that care, we urgently need a public plan of social insurance for people of all ages, including those who become disabled earlier in life. As we discussed in Chapter 7, Expanded and Improved Medicare for All (which has received hearings in the House of Representatives as H. R. 1384) will do just that.

2. Federal and state funding for LTC services.

At the federal level, enactment of Medicare for All will cover, for the first time, actual LTC services, whether provided by family caregivers in patients' homes or in other community, non-institutional settings, plus such supports as medical devices and equipment. At the state level, we can expect ongoing and expanded efforts to cover LTC services, as exemplified by Washington State's recent passage of its Long-Term Care Trust Act of 2019.

Emmanual Saez and Gabriel Zucman, economists at the University of California, Berkeley whom we met in Chapter 9, propose a progressive approach to tax reform that could readily fund the nation's needs for LTC. Their reform proposal includes these elements:

- reducing the corporate tax rate to their pre-2018 level,
- treating capital like the income tax for labor,
- setting the top marginal tax rate at 60 %, similar to the progressivity of the Truman-Eisenhower era,
- doubling of the estate tax, and
- establishing an annual wealth tax at a rate of 2 % above $50 million in wealth and 3.5 % above $1 billion.

Figure 12.1 shows how this kind of progressive reform proposal would affect taxpayers at all income levels. [13]

FIGURE 12.1

PROPOSAL RESTORING PROGRESSIVITY OF THE 1950 TAX SYSTEM

(Average tax rates by pre-tax income groups)

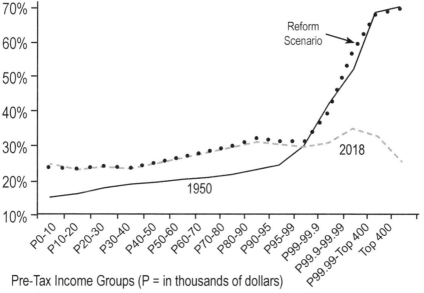

Pre-Tax Income Groups (P = in thousands of dollars)

Source: Saez, E, Zucman, G. *The Triumph of Injustice: How the Rich Dodge Taxes and How to Make Them Pay.* New York. *W. W. Norton & Company,* 2019, p. 147.

3. Fair wages and benefits.

The single biggest initiative that would start to address the nation's acute and projected shortage of long-term caregivers is to enact a $15.00/hour minimum wage. The CBO has estimated that 1.3 million American workers would be lifted out of poverty by such a change. [14] That, together with state and federal policies assuring that caregivers will also receive such benefits as paid family and medical leave, can go a long way toward recruiting and retaining an expanded caregiver workforce.

4. *A large enough caregiver workforce to meet increasing demand*

As we saw in the last chapter, the shortfall is huge—our present workforce of about 2 million direct care workers will have to grow to about 8.2 million by 2028. The challenge is actually greater, since LTC employers often struggle to fill their existing positions because of high turnover. [15]

5. *Get rid of the poverty industry*

As we saw in earlier chapters, there is an entire privatized industry in place sucking profits from the most vulnerable among us in nursing homes, assisted living and other LTC venues, even including hospices. Patients are cherry picked to increase revenues, and quality of care uniformly suffers.

In looking to the future, it is important to recall David Hatcher's statement about the poverty industry in Chapter 4:

> *Mission matters. When the poverty industry places the mission of maximizing revenue and profit over serving those in need, the vulnerable are harmed. And when the vulnerable are harmed, we are all harmed.*
>
> *We are all vulnerable. And like it or not, we are all interdependent—with each other and with our government institutions. Some of us are just more vulnerable at times than others . . . The poverty industry includes the vast combined powers of government and private enterprise. This collaboration has the capacity to do immense good, if the right goals are pursued.* [16]

6. *Training standards and certification*

Adoption of training standards and curricula along the lines of that suggested by the Paraprofessional Health Institute (PHI) (pages 149-150) will go a long way toward professionalization of direct care workers in LTC. It is also a necessary step toward certification, licensure, and new opportunities for career advancement, while also bringing more accountability to quality of personal LTC.

7. Late-in-Life Care

This is in contrast to end-of-life care. We all want to put quality of life into the equation by adding life to our years, not just years to our lives. This is more of a challenge to the boomer generation, since it has been documented to be more obese, less fit, and have more chronic conditions than their parents' generation. While it is humorous to joke that "Had I known that I would live this long, I would have taken better care of myself," that joke wears thin when major medical problems come along. Since many elderly people from their 80's on may become more frail, more subject to falls and side effects of drugs, and adverse outcomes of surgical procedures, an essential part of late-in-life care is tailoring medical care to their individual needs. Less medical care may become preferable and safer than more medical care. [17]

8. Aging in Place

As the most preferred way of aging in place—the patient's family home—this must be a leading policy target to enable that to happen as an achievable norm. As we saw in Chapter 2, there are many barriers to LTC at home, including the design of the home, the morbidities of the aging person, the availability and affordability of caregivers, and whether dementia is part of the picture. A ground level home without challenging entry steps that is wheelchair-adaptable and has an extra room for a caregiver, is a good start.

Joseph Coughlin, founder and director of MIT's AgeLab, has developed AGNES (stands for Age Gain Now Empathy System), a very heavy cumbersome suit that simulates advancing aging by making every small task very effortful. He uses this as a way to introduce seniors to what aging is likely to be like down the track when they will need help with the simplest tasks of living. [18] When evaluating the possibility of LTC at home for a person with dementia, that becomes a special challenge since patient safety will involve 24-7 care.

There are recent developments that may open up new opportunities for patients with early or moderate dementia to stay at home. These are new approaches that in some cases can delay nursing home placement, even for patients with incontinence, agitation, wandering and falling:

- Fake pets, such as a robotic kitty, can be calming and not risk a fall by walking a real dog.
- The PACE program, described in Chapter 2, which provides social opportunities, music and art activities, mild exercise, and some basic medical screening.
- *Mind at Home*, a program based at Johns Hopkins University, which sends workers to patients' homes to check out safety issues and trains caregivers to deal with dementia problems.
- *NYU Caregiver*, provides counseling sessions for family caregivers, support groups, and backup phone calls as needed. [19]

9. When a move becomes necessary

When evaluating the best location at a given time for patients needing LTC, Paula Span, author of *When the Time Comes: Families with Aging Parents Share Their Struggles and Solutions*, has developed the key questions to ask in this process. (See Appendix 1). Dementia, again, poses the most challenging evaluation of the possibilities. Under certain circumstances, a move may become necessary on an emergent basis, without preparatory lead time, as this patient's story vividly shows:

Mrs. D, 95, was growing old alone with increasingly severe cognitive deficits. Social workers had been trying but failing to improve her living conditions for more than a year. There was one member of her extended family left in the local area, but as Mrs. D. became more paranoid, she would not let her in her apartment. Her physician finally gained entrance through the cracked open door, where she found a filthy patient and apartment, a bathtub full of

*trash, pigeons in an old laundry basket, and all the win-
dows boarded up because of Mrs. D's paranoia. After a 911
call, her physician accompanied her to an ER, then on to a
nursing home.* [20]

Without a caregiver, living on one's own with advancing dementia is dangerous both for the patient and for those around him
or her.

Care vs. Cure and End-of-Life Care

If we're fortunate enough to survive accidents or serious illnesses in our middle years, the time comes later when most of us
have a number of chronic diseases, together with decreasing mobility and independence, when we need to re-evaluate when and
whether to accept traditional medical care for any given problem.
That brings to the fore the calculated equation of gain vs. risk of
poor outcomes and whether palliative care may be a better choice.

1. Palliative care

Palliative care is about improving the quality of life for people with serious illnesses or disabilities. It is focused on living as
well as possible, not on dying, as some confuse it with end-of-life
care. It includes help with how to avoid some medical care that
would have high risk of decreasing one's quality of life. It also includes symptom control, management of pain, and help with one's
daily activities. Dr. Aronson brings us this useful perspective about
palliative care:

> *Before we die, we live, and since most of us will live
> not just to old age but in it for decades, living there com-
> fortably, meaningfully, and with as much ability to do useful
> things for ourselves and others as possible matters too. Dy-
> ing as well as possible at any age requires care that takes
> into account a person's concerns, physiology, and context,
> all of which varies significantly with age.* [21]

2. End-of-life care

When it is no longer possible for a person to live on in a comfortable and meaningful way, the decision shifts to the patient's and family's preferences for end-of-life care, where it can best be provided and by whom. Most of us want to avoid what unfortunately is all too common in this country—dying in a hospital ICU, hooked up to machines, suffering, often in restraints, and sedated beyond being able to say goodbye. Hospice care may be the best answer, but the family has to explore that option carefully—many are driven by profits more than care, and some in Catholic facilities will not provide adequate pain control because of ethical and religious directives by the controlling bishops.

Maintaining a positive outlook in our declining years is obviously important, as Snoopy notes in Figure 12.2.

Figure 12.2

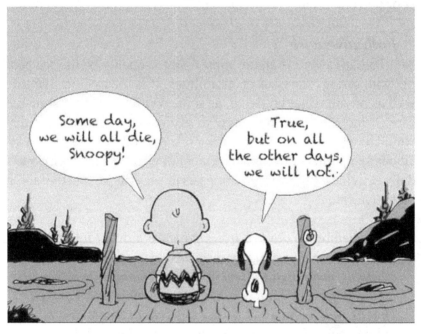

In her 2008 book, *The Gift of Years: Growing Older Gracefully*, Sister Joan Chittister points the way to better understand this process:

> We need to come to understand to the center of our souls that age is not a disease. It is a new experience in how to live life, how to milk it dry of goodness, of energy, of gratitude, of calm and quiet activity. . . One of the better gifts of growing older is that time becomes more meaningful. . . It is only in the present that we learn to live, and it is the present that is the focus of old age. . . The present finds its way into the center of our souls as it has never done before.[22]

3. The "good death" vs. bad death

A landmark 2016 study from the Sam and Rose Stein Institute for Research on Aging at the University of California San Diego School of Medicine identified the unmet needs of dying patients, as recorded by their family members and health care providers. The resulting report helps to define what we can call "successful dying," or the "good death:"

- "Preferences for the dying process (determining how death will occur; who will be there, where and when; dying in sleep; and making preparations such as advance directives and funeral arrangements)
- Pain-free status (not suffering; having pain and symptom management)
- Emotional well-being (getting emotional support; psychological comfort; having a chance to discuss the meaning of death)
- Family (having family support, family accepting of death, family prepared for death, not being a burden to the family)
- Dignity (being respected as an individual and maintaining independence)

- Life completion (saying good-bye, feeling that life was well lived, and accepting imminent death)
- Religiosity/spirituality (religious or spiritual comfort; faith; meeting with clergy)
- Treatment preferences (not prolonging life, a belief that all available treatments were used; control of treatment; accessing euthanasia/physician assisted death)
- Quality of life, (living life as usual; maintaining hope, pleasure, gratitude, feeling life is worth living)
- Relationship with health care provider (having trust in and gaining support and comfort from physicians and nurses; having a physician who is comfortable with death and dying; being able to discuss spiritual beliefs or fears with a physician)
- Other (recognition of culture; experiencing physical touch; being with pets; considering health care costs)" [23]

Not surprisingly, this report found that many of these criteria were commonly not met. Dr. Dilip Jeste, the lead researcher, said later that "For a dying person, the concerns seem to be more existential and psychological and less physical." [24]

There are still systemic barriers to the "good death" that end up with 'bad deaths' being far more common. Many physicians are still uncomfortable in discussing realistic prognoses and options for end-of-life care. [25] While older Americans say they want to die at home, 75 percent of people dying in hospitals are over age 65. [26] Catholic hospitals will not refer dying patients to Compassion and Choices. Advance directives are often not available or followed. Physician-assisted death is legal in nine states, but few Americans actually choose it. [27]

Conclusion

This is not an ending at the end of this book. Instead, it is hopefully one small step toward an expanded dialogue that can lead to a much better and responsive system for personal, affordable, long term care for the common good, not for corporate profits.

Isn't care of so many tens of millions of elderly and other persons with disabilities and/or dementia worth investing in their care, in a country where they have contributed for so many years, and are now grandparents and even great grandparents of new generations of Americans? Is this an America that values earlier generations, treasures and builds on the past, or a country only interested in dollars and the immediate future?

Robert Reich, Ph.D., professor of public policy at the University of California Berkeley and author of the excellent 2018 book, *The Common Good,* helps us to answer this fundamental question:

> *The common good consists of our shared values about what we owe one another as citizens who are bound together in the same society—the norms we voluntarily abide by, and the ideals we seek to achieve. . . . A concern for the common good is a moral attitude. It recognizes that we're all in it together.* [28]

Does that observation become a moral imperative, since we all age, encounter adversities along the way, often need long-term care toward the end, and finally die either a good or bad death?! If it does, do we have enough political will to address the personal and national crisis in our current non-system of long-term care in this country?

References

1. Kleinman, A. Treating disease is no substitute for caring for the ill. *Wall Street Journal*, November 30-December 1, 2019: C3.
2. Aronson, L. *Elderhood: Redefining Aging, Transforming Medicine, Reimagining Life.* New York. *Bloomsbury Publishing*, 2019, p. 270.
3. Carstensen, LL. We need a major redesign of life. *The Washington Post*, November 29, 2019.
4. Graham, J. A doctor speaks out about ageism in medicine. *Kaiser Health News,* May 30, 2019.

5.   Gopnik, A. Younger longer: Can the infirmities of aging be postponed? *The New Yorker*, May 20, 2019, p. 36.

6.   Aronson, L, as quoted by Graham, J. A doctor speaks out about ageism in medicine. *Kaiser Health News*, May 30, 2019.

7.   Larson, EB, DeClaire, J. *Enlightened Aging: Building Resilience for a Long, Active Life*. New York. *Rowman & Littlefield*, 2017, p. 19.

8.   Horovitz, B. Why your perception of 'old' changes as you age. *Kaiser Health News*, June 11, 2019.

9.   Rousseau, MC et al. Quality of life in patients with locked-in syndrome: Evolution over a 6-year period. *Orphanet Journal of Rare Diseases* 10.88, 2015.

10. Powell, T. *Dementia Reimagined: Building a Life of Joy and Dignity from Beginning to End*. New York. *Penguin Random House*, 2019, p. 214.

11. Heumann, J., as quoted by LaSpina, N. *Such a Pretty Girl: A Story of Struggle, Empowerment and Disability Pride*. New York. *New Village Press*, 2019.

12. Ibid # 9, pp. 221-222.

13. Saez, E, Zucman, G. *The Triumph of Injustice: How the Rich Dodge Taxes and How to Make Them Pay*. New York. *W. W. Norton & Company*, 2019, p. 147.

14.   Morath, E. CBO sees $15 pay as mixed bag for workers. *Wall Street Journal*, July 9, 2019: A2.

15. Campbell, S., personal communication. 8.2 million direct care jobs will need to be filled by 2028. PHI. Paraprofessional Health Institute National, October, 2019.

16. Hatcher, DL. *The Poverty Industry: The Exploitation of America's Most Vulnerable Citizens*. New York. *New York University Press*, 2016, p. 221.

17. Ibid # 6, p. 161-162, 176.

18. Ibid # 4.

19. Powell, T. New hopes for dementia care. *Wall Street Journal,* April 13-14, 2019.

20. Ibid # 10, pp. 203-204.

21. Ibid # 2, p. 370.

22. Chittister, J. *The Gift of Years: Growing Older Gracefully*, Katonah, New York. BlueBridge, 2008: pp. 54, 202-203.

23. Meier, EA et al. Defining a Good Death (Successful Dying): Literature Review and a Call for Research and Public Dialogue. *American Journal of Geriatric Psychiatry* 24 (4): 261-271, 2016.)

24. Netburn, D, What does it mean to have a good death? *Los Angeles Times,* April 1, 2016.

25. Aleccia, JN. Never say 'die': Why so many doctors won't break bad news. *Kaiser Health News*, June 12, 2019.
26. National Center for Health Statistics. Trends in Inpatient Hospital Deaths: National Hospital Discharge Survey, 2000-2010. Centers for Disease Control and Prevention.
27. Span, P. Aid in dying soon will be available to more Americans. Few will choose it. *New York Times*, July 8, 2019.
28. Reich, R. *The Common Good*. New York. *Alfred A Knopf*. 2018, p. 18.

SOME QUESTIONS TO CONSIDER IN SELECTING LONG-TERM CARE SETTINGS

Reprinted with permission from Paula Span, author of *When the Time Comes: Families With Aging Parents Share Their Struggles and Solutions*, New York, *Springboard Press*, 2009

HOME CARE

What tasks does your parent need help with in order to remain in her home? How many of the ADLs—activities of daily living like bathing, dressing, and eating—will she need assistance with? What about the IADLs—instrumental activities of daily living, meaning household chores like preparing meals, housecleaning, and money management?

Does your parent have a social network and community connections that remain important? Is she engaged with friends and neighbors, a religious congregation, volunteer projects, or civic groups? Those ties can be a strong impetus to stay put.

Can she move about her community for shopping, medical appointments, and recreation? Can friends, volunteers, local agencies, or paid helpers provide enough transportation to prevent isolation?

Is your parent's home safe and functional for a senior with health problems or disabilities? Can it be adapted by installing a shower bench, grab bars, toilet risers? Is it practical to build a wheelchair ramp if one's required, to widen doorways or put in a stair lift?

How much paid home care will be sufficient to allow her to age in place? A few hours of homemaker assistance daily? Home health aides day and night? Skilled nursing care?

Can she or the family put that much help in place, and pay for it privately? Can publicly funded programs—through Medicaid, city and state programs, or local charities—help make home care affordable?

Is your parent sociable and communicative enough to form relationships with paid caregivers? Does she have behavioral problems, such as those caused by dementia, that will make it difficult for them to help her, and difficult for her to retain them?

Will she be able to reliably report how her caregivers are working out, what problems have arisen, whether she's happy with the arrangement? Will you or other family members be able to drop in to monitor her care?

SHARING A HOUSEHOLD

Can your parent function independently in your home? Will he be able to manage most of his personal care? Pitch in with some household duties? Or will he need not only a room, meals, and transportation but also help with ADLs—activities of daily living like bathing or dressing?

Can you retrofit your home, or sections of it, to make it safe for an elderly person with health problems or disabilities? Will your parent be secure on the stairs and in the bathroom?

How important is privacy, and can you adapt your home to provide it? Will sharing a bathroom, or a single television set or phone line, be problematic? Will household noises disturb your parent? Will his waking up at night or watching TV at high volume disturb you?

If you're working, will your parent spend his days alone? Will that be risky, or isolating? Are there local senior centers or adult day programs that can provide him with companionship, meals, perhaps health monitoring, during the day?

Have you discussed with other family members the changes your parent's move into your household will bring? The ways it may impact your schedules and routines, your work and school and social lives? Your finances?

If your parent is unable to be home alone for more than a few hours, can you arrange for occasional respite care, so that you can take a business trip, have a weekend away, plan a vacation?

Do you and your parent have a history of enjoying time together, discussing problems openly, reaching compromises? Will your personalities fit amicably under one roof?

Can siblings or other family members share the responsibilities, even if your parent is living in your household? Can they stay in your home while you're away, take your parent on regular outings, or help pay out-of-pocket costs?

ASSISTED LIVING

Does your parent need help with housekeeping, meal preparation and such activities of daily living as bathing, dressing, and remembering medications? Assisted living is primarily designed for seniors requiring this level of assistance.

Is she otherwise able to live comfortably in her own room or small apartment? Can she feed herself? Use a toilet or manage her own incontinence garments? If not, your parent may need more help and supervision than most assisted living residences provide.

Is she mobile enough, with a cane, walker, or wheelchair, to go to and from the dining room and to participate in activities and outings?

Does she require vigilant daily health monitoring (of blood glucose levels, for instance) or regular skilled nursing care? Most assisted living facilities don't provide such services, even if there is a nurse on the staff.

Can your parent or family afford steep monthly fees? In most cases, assisted living residents pay privately. But Medicaid will pay part of the tab in some states, and some facilities offer subsidized apartments; have you looked into such arrangements?

Can family members, trusted friends, or a geriatric care manager visit your parent weekly or more often, not only to spend time will her but to monitor her care? Can they come on varying days and at odd times?

Is your parent social enough to form relationships with staffers and friendships with fellow residents? Is she adaptable enough for a group residence?

NURSING HOMES

Does your parent need help with almost all activities, including moving around his room and eating meals? Does he need two helpers in order to safely take a shower or use a toilet? A nursing home is the most likely facility to provide this much assistance.

Does he require hour-by-hour monitoring and nursing care, during the day and at night—more assistance than most families can afford to hire at home and more than most assisted living facilities offer?

Does he need physical or occupational therapy, or help from a social worker? Nursing homes generally have such specialized care available onsite; other facilities may not.

Has he exhausted his assets, or will he soon, so that he will be eligible for Medicaid? Skilled nursing facilities are the only long-term care option that Medicaid will pay for regardless of the state your parent lives in; coverage for other alternatives, like home care or assisted living, varies from state to state.

Can family members, trusted friends, or a geriatric care manager check on your parent regularly, sometimes at odd hours, to be sure he is receiving the care he needs? Can you locate a nursing home with a family council, so that family members can support one another and communicate with administrators as a group?

HOSPICE CARE

Has your parent been diagnosed with a terminal disease? Will a physician certify that the disease, untreated, is likely to result in death within six months? That's what hospice eligibility requires.

Do your parent and family understand what hospice care entails? Do they know that it's an approach to the end of life, rather than a place, although a few hospice organizations do offer residences? That it aims to help patients end their lives at home?

Is your parent ready, after discussion with family members, health care providers, and hospice staff, to exchange procedures meant to cure illness for palliative care that instead provides comfort and pain management? Hospice patients need not reject all medical care, but the goals of care shift.

Would your parent prefer to die, not in a hospital, but in her own home, in a family member's home, or in the place she now calls home, an assisted living facility or nursing home?

As she nears the end of her life, would a team—including nurses, a social worker, home care aides, a chaplain—be helpful to her and to the family? Does the family want assistance with keeping the patient comfortable, understanding her status, meeting her emotional and spiritual needs? This is the hospice approach.

Are there caregivers, either family members or employees, who can be with your parent as she needs more help? Hospice patients can't live alone as they decline and can no longer care for themselves. Though hospice staffers can always be summoned in case of emergencies, they can't be with patients around the clock.

Do family members want support for themselves through this transition, as well as for their parent? Hospices regard the family, not the patient alone, as their clients.

APPENDIX 2

RECOMMENDED READING

Aronson, Louise. *Elderhood: Redefining Aging, Transforming Medicine, Reimagining Life.* New York, NY. *Bloomsbury Publishing*, 2019.

Byock, I. *Dying Well: The Prospect for Growth at the End of Life*, New York, NY, *Riverhead Books*, 1997.

Chittister, J. *The Gift of Years: Growing Older Gracefully.* Katonah, New York. *BlueBridge*, 2008.

Geyman, J. *Souls on a Walk: An Enduring Love Story Unbroken by Alzheimer's.* Friday Harbor, WA. *Copernicus Healthcare*, 2012.

Gleckman, H. *Caring for Our Parents: Inspiring Stories of Families Seeking New Solutions to America's Most Urgent Crisis.* New York, NY. *St. Martin's Press*, 2009.

Harrold, JK, Lynn, J. (Eds) *A Good Dying: Shaping Health Care for the Last Months of Life*. New York, NY. *The Hawarth Press, Inc*, 1998.

Hatcher, DL. *The Poverty Industry: The Exploitation of America's Most Vulnerable Citizens.* New York, NY. *New York University Press*, 2016.

Jacoby, S. *Never Say Die: The Myth and Marketing of the New Old Age. Pantheon Books*, New York, 2011.

Kleinman, A. T*he Soul of Care: The Moral Education of a Husband and Doctor.* New York. *Penguin Random House*, 2019.

Larson, WB, DeClaire, J. *Enlightened Aging: Building Resilience for a Long, Active Life*. New York, NY. *Rowman & Littlefield*, 2017.

LaSpina, N. *Such a Pretty Girl: A Story of Struggle, Empowerment, and Disability Pride*. New York. *New Village Press*, 2019.

Miller, BJ, Berger, S. *A Beginner's Guide to the End: Practical Advice for Living Life and Facing Death.* New York. *Simon & Schuster*, 2019.

Moss, H. *The 2030 Caregiving Crisis: A Heavy Burden for Boomer Children*, Bronx, NY. *Henry Moss*, 2015.

Powell, T. *Dementia Reimagined: Building a Life of Joy and Dignity from Beginning to End.* New York, NY. *Penguin Random House*, 2019.

Span, P. *When the Time Comes: Families with Aging Parents Share their Struggles and Solutions*, New York, NY. *Springboard*, 2009.

APPENDIX 3

USEFUL RESOURCES

NATIONAL LONG-TERM CARE ORGANIZATIONS

Administration for Community Living
330 C St. SW
Washington, D.C. 20201
202-401-4634
800-677-1116 (to find local resources)

Alzheimer's Association
225 N. Michigan Avenue, 17th Floor,
Chicago, IL 60601-7633
800-272-3900
www.alz.org

American Association of Retired People (AARP)
601 E Street NW,
Washington, DC 20049
888-OUR-AARP
www.aarp.org/caregiving

Americans Disabled Attendant Programs Today (ADAPT)
Campus Box 12345
Durham, NC 27708-0680
919-660-1234

Assisted Living Association of America
  1650 King Street, Suite 602
  Alexandria, VA 22314-2747
  703-894-1805
  www.alfa.org

Center for Excellence in Assisted Living (CEAL)
  1120 20th Street NW, Suite 750
  Washington, DC, 20036-3441
  202-216-9623
  info@theceal.org

Centers for Medicare and Medicaid Services (CMS)
  Resource for LTC and advance directive planning through
  medicare.gov
  1-800-633-4227
  Medicare Contact Center Operations
  P. O. Box 1270
  Lawrence, KS 66044

Compassion & Choices
  Resource for advance directives, including dementia
  provision and Physician Orders for Life Sustaining
  Treatment (POLST)
  101 SW Madison Street, # 8009
  Portland, OR 97207
  800-247-7421

Consortium for Citizens with Disabilities
  820 First Street NE, Suite 740
  Washington, DC 20002
  202-567-3516
  Info@c-c-d.org

Consumer Consortium on Assisted Living
2342 Oak Street,
Falls Church, VA 22046
703-533-8121
www.ccal.org

Disabled in Action
P. O. Box 30954
Port Authority Station
New York, NY, 10011-0109
718-261-3737

Family Caregiver Alliance
180 Montgomery Street, Suite 1100
San Francisco, CA 94104
88-445-8106
www.caregiver.org

Gerontological Society of America
1220 L Street NW, Suite 901
Washington, DC 20005
201-842-1275

Hospice Association of America
228 Seventh Street SE
Washington, DC 20003
202-547-7424

Long-Term Care Nurses Association
1029 South Fourth Street
Springfield, IL 62703-2224
217-528-6455
800-252-8988

National Academy of Social Insurance
  Designing Universal Family Care
  Washington, D. C.
  nasi@nasi.org
  202-452-8111

National Alliance for Caregiving
  4720 Montgomery Lane, 5th Floor
  Bethesda, MD 20814
  301-718-8444
  www.caregiving.org

National Association for Home Care and Hospice
  228 Seventh Street, SE
  Washington, D.C. 20003
  202-547-7424

National Center for Assisted Living
  1201 L Street NW,
  Washington, DC 20005
  202-842-4444
  www.ncal.org

National Center on Elder Abuse
  1201 15th Street NW, Suite 350
  Washington, DC 20005
  202-898-2586

NCCNHR. National Citizens' Coalition
  for Nursing Home Reform
  1828 L Street NW, Suite 801,
  Washington, DC 20036
  202-332-2275
  www.nccnhr.org

National Family Caregivers Association
    10400 Connecticut Avenue, Suite 500
    Kensington, MD 20895
    800-896-3650
    www.nfcacares.org

National Hospice and Palliative Care Organization
    1731 King Street, Suite 100,
    Alexandria, VA 22314
    800-658-8898
    www.nhpco.org

National Nurses United
    8455 Colesville Road, Suite 1100
    Silver Spring, MD 20910
    240-235-2000
    info@nationalnursesunited.org

Paraprofessional Healthcare Institute (PHI)
    400 East Fordham Road, 11th Floor
    Bronx, NY 10458
    718-402-7766
    info@PHInational.org

Physicians for a National Health Program (PNHP)
    29 E. Madison Street, Suite 1412
    Chicago, IL 60602
    312-782-6006
    info@pnhp.org

Programs of All Inclusive Care of the Elderly (PACE)
    National PACE Association
    675 North Washington St., Suite 300
    Alexandria, VA 22314

Public Citizen
  215 Pennsylvania Ave. SE
  Washington, DC 20003
  202-546-4996

U. S. Department of Health and Human Services
  Resource for tools and links for LTC planning, including
    LTC Pathfinder
  LongTermCare.gov

DISCUSSION QUESTIONS

1. What would you do when a family member could take care of other members of the family but their own circumstances would suffer?

These two stories (referenced in Chapter 2) from family caregivers raise many questions, often not asked or answered, as they cope with caring for parents or other family members when they can no longer care for themselves.

Alexis Baden-Mayer, now 45, moved with her husband and two children three years ago to take care of her parents at their home in Alexandria, Virginia. They put their own home on AirBnB to make the move when her mother developed Alzheimer's disease and was no longer able to care for her father with heart failure. In so doing, Alexis joined the army of some 34 million family caregivers, mostly women, providing uncompensated care to frail elderly family members in the U. S. As she says now, a frank conversation with her husband (not held in these blunt terms) would (or should?) have been: "What do you think about living with my parents for about ten years while their health declines and they die?"

Mrs. EF, 64, was working as a home health aide for seniors near San Ysidro, California, when she had to give up her job to provide the same care for her husband when she was recovering from triple bypass surgery. His health then declined as he developed vascular dementia with erratic

behavior that caused her to fall and injure her back. He
was admitted to one nursing home but later discharged because of his behavior. The local hospital was unable to find
another place for him, so Maria brought him back home
under her care.

Questions for discussion:

1. If you were Alexis, what conversation would you
   have had with her husband and children before moving in with her parents?
2. What ethical issues are raised by these circumstances
   that may be helpful to some family members but det-
   rimental to others?
3. How can such decisions be reached while preserving
   the dignity and best interests of all members of the
   family?
4. If you were Maria, could you have done anything
   else, and what new challenges is she likely to face by
   making this decision?
5. After reading this book and seeing all the system
   problems facing long-term care in this country, what
   kind of system reform would you favor?

2. Genetic testing for Alzheimer's disease.

As you have seen in this book, there is no effective treatment
yet for Alzheimer's disease. While there is also no way to prevent
it, there is much activity in trying to develop genetic testing to
identify one's future risk of developing the disease. At this stage,
however, genetic testing for Alzheimer's is still controversial
among experts, may not be of predictive value, and may raise hurt-
ful anxieties for people and their families. These tests are being
sold and marketed on line by such companies as *23andMe*, as this
person's story illustrates:

*Theresa Braymer, 59, a retired Navy commander liv-
ing in the Denver area, has no family history of Alzheimer's
but tested positive for a gene variant that might predict its
future onset. The use of this testing is still controversial, but
genetic testing is being marketed widely, so many people
will get results like this and have to decide how to assess
them for themselves.* [1]

1. Reddy, S. Are you at greater risk of Alzheimer's? *Wall Street Journal*, July 16, 2019: A10.

Questions for group discussion:

1. Given the lack of effective prevention or treatment of Alzheimer's disease, would you want to get a gene test?

2. If you did choose to be tested, what would you do if you
   received this kind of result?

3. These further questions, raised in my 2012 book, *Souls on
   a Walk: An Enduring Love Story Unbroken by Alzheimer's,*
   may also be of interest for group discussion:

   a. If you are faced with the care of your spouse or family
      member with Alzheimer's, what new life plan would
      you consider for yourself and your family?

   b. If you had to move to care for a family member with
      Alzheimer's, where would you go, and how would
      the move impact your own life?

D

I

immigrants
    discrimination, 108, 109 (Fig. 8.2)
    under Trump administration, 109, 152
    individual mandate repeal, 115
in-patient care costs, 36
insurance
    employer-sponsored history 92
    job-based, 92
    lack, 1
    Los Angeles Times analysis, 92
    loss in nursing home, 96
    private and multi-payer, 78, 81, 97
    taxpayer costs, inflated, 129

J

Jayapal Pramila, single-payer bill, 131
Jacobs, Alice (patient history story), 117
Jeste, Dr. Dilip, 172
Johnson, Lyndon, President, 78

K

Kaiser Family Foundation study of Medicare and Social Security (quote), 40
Kaiser Health Ne ws (KHN), 36, 55, 57
    employer-sponsored health insurance, 38
    federal Medicare overpayments, 82 (Fig. 6.2)
    scams/fraud 55, 57,Äî58
Kennedy, Senator Ted, 69
King, Rev. Dr. Martin Luther (in quote), 121
King, Theresa story of LTC, 103-104
Kleinman, M.D. (quote), 159
Kuttner, Robert, *Everything for Sale* (quote), 116

L

LaGuardia, New York City Mayor, quote) 159
Larson, Dr. Eric, 150, *Enlightened Aging* book, 161-162
Lederman, Dr. Leon example, 43
Life Alert, 29
Life Care Centers of America, closure, 54-55
    employer-sponsored health insurance, 38

M

N

O

P

Q

R

T

Tacrine approval for Alzheimer's disease, 69
taxes
  restoring progressivity, 165 (Fig. 12.1)
  on wealthy, 118, 134
Tax Equity and Fiscal Responsibility Act, 78-79
tax rates, 115 (Fig. 9.1), 115
Theoharis, Liz, 121 (quote), 121
total care hours, non-institutional, 65
training standards and certification, 166
Trigg, Roxanne, home health aide (quote), 101-102
Trump, President, and Trump administration
  attempts to repeal ACA and Medicaid, 114, 116
  budgets and budget cuts, 115, 116, 127
  caregiver LTC, recruitment, 109
  "Great plan," 130
  immigrants, skilled decrease, and zero-tolerance policies, 109, 152
  multi-payer bureaucracy, 135
  nursing homes, 56
  presidency and problems, 80, 81, 98
  tax bill and policies, 117, 118, 119
Twain, Mark (quote), 120
Twenty "20-80 rule, 97

U

unaffordability of long-term care, 1
underinsured U.S. adults not affording care, 127
uninsured in 2017, 139
unionization, lack of political power, 109-110, 109
UnitedHealth Group, 76
universal coverage, 15, 128, 132
Universal Family Care, Designing, 154
U.S. Bureau of Labor Statistics, home care wages, 147
U.S. Census Bureau and Statistia (Fig. 1.1), 6
U.S. Department of Labor
  growing, 105
  for home health care workers, 104, 153
U.S. health care system, 1, 2
  financing, 128
  ownership, 80 (Fig. 6.1)
U.S. population, tripling by 2050, 66
U.S. workers leaving jobs (quit rate), 137

V

Vanderbilt, Cornelius, 120
Verma, Seema, CMS administrator, 42
Village Movement (Beacon Hill originator), 27

W

wage, minimal, favor doubling, 134
Wall Street, 71
    bull market, 38
    investors / S & P 500, 35, 53, 113
    Warren, Sen. Elizabeth, 117
Washington Post article on doubling of for-profit hospices, 56
Washington State Long-term Care Trust Act of 2019, 155
wealth, 117
women, 15
    dementia, 102
    home health care, 153
    vs. male spending (quote), 40
Woodlander, Dr. 139 (quote)
Wylie, David and Sally quote because of insurance loss, 95

Z

Zucman, Gabriel 119 (book quote), 164

About The Author

John Geyman, M.D. is professor emeritus of Family Medicine at the University of Washington School of Medicine in Seattle, where he served as Chairman of the Department of Family Medicine from 1976 to 1990. As a family physician with over 21 years in academic medicine, he also practiced in rural communities for 13 years. He was the founding editor of *The Journal of Family Practice* (1973 to 1990) and the editor of *The Journal of the American Board of Family Medicine* from

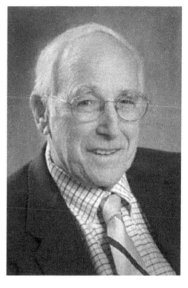

1990 to 2003. Since 1990 he has been involved with research and writing on health policy and health care reform.

His most recent books are *Struggling and Dying under TrumpCare: How We Can Fix this Fiasco* (2019) and a pamphlet, *Common Sense: The Case For and Against Medicare for All, Leading Issue in the 2020 Elections* (2019); *TrumpCare: Lies, Broken Promises, How It Is Failing, and What Should Be Done?* (2018), and a pamphlet, *Common Sense: U. S. Health Care at a Crossroads in the 2018 Congress*, (2018), and *Crisis in U. S. Health Care: Corporate Power vs. The Common Good* (2017), *Common Sense about Health Care Reform in America* (pamphlet, 2017).

Dr. Geyman founded his own small, independent publishing firm, Copernicus Healthcare about ten years ago, which has published such books as *Everybody In Nobody Out: Memoirs of a*

Rebel Without a Pause by Dr. Quentin Young (2013) and *Health, Medicine and Justice: Designing a Fair and Equitable Healthcare System* by Dr. Joshua Freeman (2015). (www.copernicus-health-care.org)

Dr. Geyman is a member of the National Academy of Medicine (formerly the Institute of Medicine), and served as the president of Physicians for a National Health Program from 2005 to 2007.

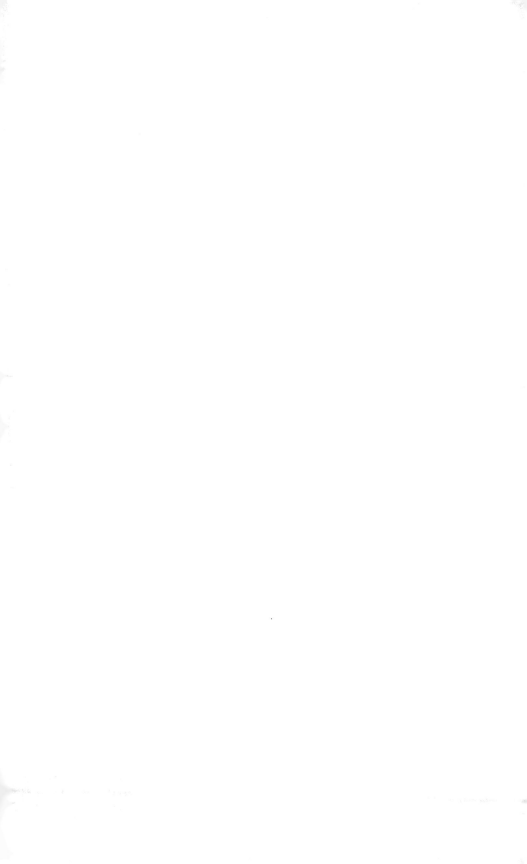

CPSIA information can be obtained
at www.ICGtesting.com
Printed in the USA
BVHW071401140120
569037BV00002B/5/P